eat to your heart's content

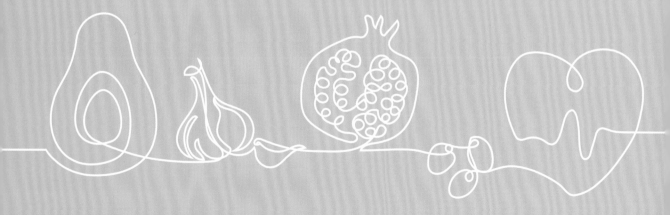

eat to your heart's content

Sat Bains

Recipes to improve your heart health
from a Michelin Star Chef

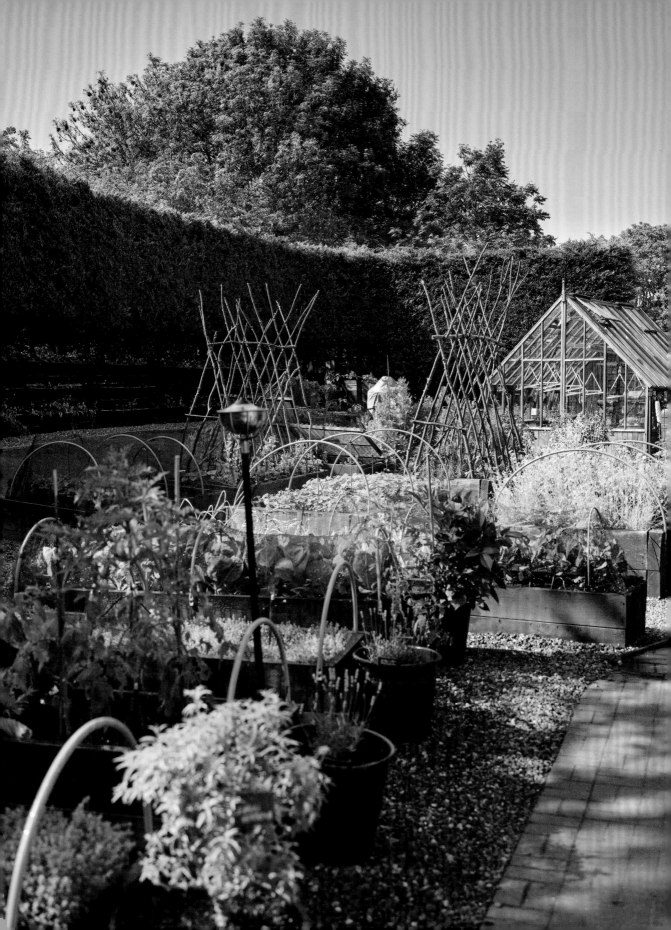

Contents

Introduction | Sat Bains . . . 7

Getting started . . . 12

Heart-healthy eating | Dr Neil Williams . . . 16

1   **Eggs** . . . 22

2   **Salads** . . . 38

3   **Vegetables** . . . 60

4   **Fish** . . . 90

5   **Meat** . . . 114

6   **Soups, sauces, pickles and broths** . . . 142

7   **Smoothies, snacks and breads** . . . 158

8   **Sweet things** . . . 170

Index . . . 186

Acknowledgements . . . 191

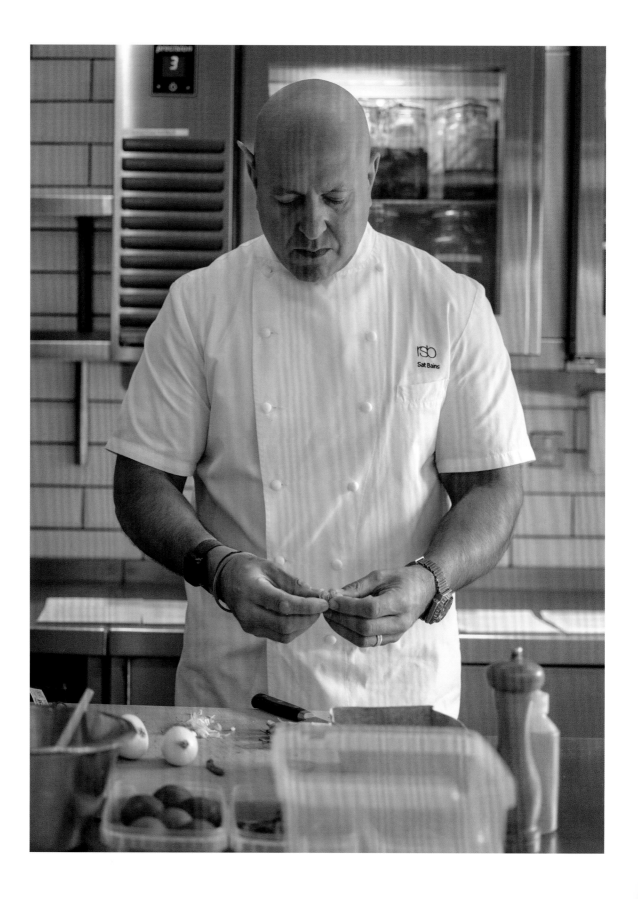

introduction

Sat Bains

It was March 2020. Lockdown was easing a little, prior to this I was enjoying a life filled with fun, laughter, love, great food, great wine and hard work, and believed I had achieved a really good work–life balance. Then, out of nowhere, I had a heart attack.

I had just turned 50.

I'm a fit guy, have done weight training since I was 14, and have held a gym membership for as long as I can remember, so it was a shock to find myself in an ambulance being taken to A&E. I'm here to tell you, though, that it is possible to make a recovery. I am a heart attack survivor.

On the day it happened, I was home doing a fitness routine in the garden with Nick Warren – my trainer for the last several years – when, 20 minutes in, I felt a pain in my left pectoral. I thought it was muscular, as I was doing some heavy weights, and said to Nick, 'Bloody hell, it's a hard one today!' I pushed through until I finished the session, thinking nothing more of it apart from my deep hatred towards Nick at the end of each session ha ha ha . . . Check him out on Insta @n_gymstarr. I showered, ate, then headed to the supermarket with Amanda, my wife, an outing we followed with a walk in the park. Our regular lockdown routine, in fact. But at the park I lacked energy and felt tired, not like me at all.

I like to monitor my fitness progress and wear a WHOOP strap. One of its functions is to register your heart rate. Worryingly, it was sporadic. The pain was becoming more intense and I was increasingly irritable. Pain was creeping along my left jawline, behind my eye socket and slowly working down my shoulder. Classic signs, I now realize, of a heart attack. By the time I got home I was aware that something definitely wasn't right, so I called 999. An ambulance arrived, blue lights flashing - the full works - quickly followed by more paramedics. There were more people in the house than we'd seen in the whole of lockdown!

Anyone who has had a heart attack will be familiar with what happened next. I was attached to an ECG and given a squirt of nitroglycerine under my tongue to open up my capillaries and allow my blood to flow more freely. On arrival at Nottingham City Hospital, I was given an angiogram - a tube that passes through an artery in the wrist to get to the heart, through which dye is injected into the coronary arteries, allowing doctors to identify the blockage causing the heart attack. Mine showed that I had a massive blood clot preventing the normal flow of blood to the heart.

After the angiogram I was given blood thinners, to dilute the clot. With blood clots, though, you've got to be super careful. When being dissolved, pieces can break off and get carried to the brain, resulting in a stroke. In my naivety, I thought that would be it, and I'd be back home after a couple days.

Once the thinners had done their job, though, there were more tests. A second angiogram, X-rays, an MRI and another ECG. By now doctors realized that I had severe narrowing at the top of my left coronary artery just as it divided into its two main branches, something that could not be easily fixed by stents. It would require major surgery to put it right. I clearly wasn't going home anytime soon.

Initially, we considered three options. I could travel to London for keyhole surgery, something that was quickly discounted as I was too ill to move. Alternatively, I could have open-heart surgery. The third option I can't remember, to be honest with you. Once I was settled in a bed, I met the doctors and surgeons, all of whom said the same thing, which was that they were quite surprised I was still alive. The severity of the heart attack and the size of the clot 'should have killed me that morning'. Not surprisingly, it was decided an operation couldn't wait.

I was fit and otherwise healthy so the best option was for me to have an open-heart triple bypass, the beating heart method, where your heart continues to function and you don't go on a ventilator as it allows for a better recovery. The anaesthetist talked me through what would happen. An artery would be taken from my arm to use reuse in my chest. My chest plate would be cut open, my ribs broken, and I'd be sliced straight down the middle. Quite a shock to hear someone say that to you!

We were still in the midst of COVID so I was surprised when they asked if Amanda was coming to see me. They suggested I call her. It was then that I knew how serious it all was. Amanda came, we chatted, we cried. I was trying to be upbeat, and to see her so upset definitely tested my mental resolve, but I felt strong. I went into theatre at 10.30am and regained consciousness around 9pm. Amanda had been calling and checking throughout so when I came round and was able to speak to her, it was probably the most relieved both of us have ever felt. The surgeon, Mr Naik, is probably one of the best in the country and I feel truly blessed. He saved my life.

There's no getting away, though, from the fact that it was major surgery, and to say I was quite ill afterward is an understatement. For a guy who has spent most of his life being strong, both mentally and physically, I found the weeks and months that followed really testing. I was unable to take even a few steps and was in a lot of pain. I couldn't sleep on my sides as my chest was wired and stitched closed. I was exhausted.

Hospital was hard for me, and I was very much out of my comfort zone. I am someone who normally has control of his day-to-day life and having to relinquish this was very difficult. My days were spent watching motivational videos, listening to podcasts, trying to keep my mind occupied. It was the first time in my life I could do nothing! The food wasn't great, either, mainly processed foods, chips and toast, and as a result I had no appetite. The hospital staff, though, from the surgeons to the nurses, were incredible; they helped me daily to understand what was going on and I will be forever grateful to them for that.

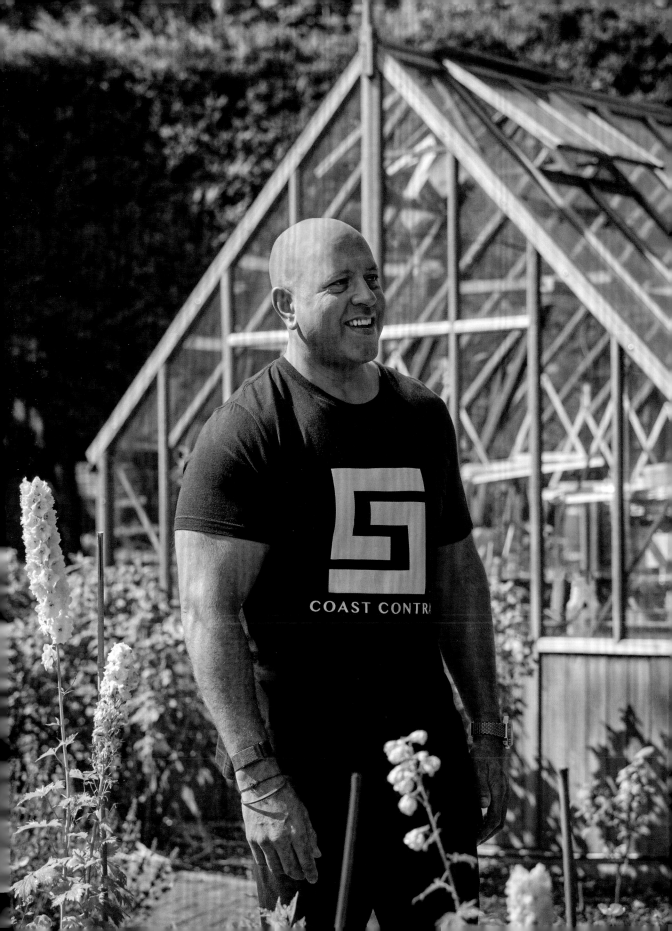

Coming out of hospital was a relief but also very difficult. I had to be monitored at home and couldn't be left alone. Amanda had to juggle the business during a global pandemic and at the same time care for me. I will never know where she got the strength from, but she did, and I love her the more for it. She has been the most incredible person in my life and one of the major factors in my speedy recovery.

I had family and friends on a rota system. Being waited on hand and foot really didn't suit me, and I hated every minute, but I shut up and worked on my recovery. I had to wear compression socks for the first six weeks after surgery. If you've ever had to wear them, you will know that they are incredibly difficult to put on. If I'd had to do it myself it probably would have given me another heart attack. So, every day, twice a day, Amanda would take them off and cream my feet and put them back on, we had so much fun. Ha ha. Not.

Just walking upstairs was a major event, it took me ages. Fortunately, we have a toilet downstairs (sit down wees only!), which meant I didn't have to go far when I got up off the sofa. Even so, I would feel dizzy from the rush of blood as I stood up, and the medication took some time to get used to. But I persevered and got up every two hours to walk around the table as advised by my surgeon.

I was kept strong mentally by my daily chats with my good friend Michael Mason. A machine of a man, he kept me focused and I could share my inner thoughts and motivation with him. I thank him so much for being there for me. Check him out on Insta @masonsurvival.

From talking to Michael I knew I had to put my time at home to good use if I was to recover from this very invasive surgery. My appetite was gone, and all I wanted to eat were very small portions of bland, boring but 'healthy' food around five times a day. I'd lost 17kg and looked gaunt. I had to improve – and vary – my nutrition. My thoughts went straight to Mediterranean and Japanese diets. I already knew the health benefits of lots of fish, lean meats, vegetables, yams, dashi, seaweed and green teas and thought this could be the way forward.

So, I spoke to Dr Neil Williams, Senior Lecturer in Exercise Physiology and Nutrition at Nottingham Trent University. He was someone who had helped me in the past when I went to Everest base camp – he'd even allowed me to use the altitude chamber at the university for my training. But that's a story for another time.

With Neil's guidance, I began to devise weekly heart-healthy menus, measuring all my foods down to the last gram, that suited my needs for recovery and strength, but still put the onus on flavour. Flavour has been an obsession for my entire career and I was determined not to sacrifice it. It's why I decided to write this book, as I realized there was a lack of resource for anyone who wants flavoursome, heart-healthy, accessible food that makes you feel good and strong.

My diet now consists of lean protein and a mix of legumes, vegetables and fruits, as well as good fats such as avocado, nuts and olive oil. It's a diet that anyone can follow as there's lots of room to manoeuvre, where you can change the main protein source to one that suits you.

I have had several check-ups, including ones at three and nine months since my heart attack, and I've passed them all with flying colours. My consultant, Dr Varcoe, has been hugely impressed by my recovery and has taken me off a few meds along the way. The saving factor for me was my fitness. It was the only reason I am still standing. I still train most days, take regular 5k walks, do Krav Maga every Saturday morning and do functional training, spin classes and stretching. I am probably a little less intense in my training now, though, and I make sure it is more varied.

I wanted to share this journey with you so you understand the history of what happened to me. I wanted, also, to emphasize that eating decent, healthy food doesn't mean you need to compromise on flavour. I've used the experience I've gained over more than three decades of being a chef to create the recipes in this book – all of which use normal, accessible ingredients – and to make them exciting by incorporating spices, a splash of soy, a drizzle of fruity olive oil, fresh herbs and seasonings.

The recipes are accompanied by Dr Neil Williams's incredibly valuable nutritional tips, which will help to guide you in your choices. Insightful and succinct, his words explain the science without being too technical. His Top 10 Heart-healthy Foods on page 17 should be on every fridge as guidance for us all.

What I didn't want to do was write a preachy, unattainable 'diet' book that would end up gathering dust on a shelf. I still enjoy the odd fish and chips, a juicy steak, red wine and a pizza. We all, on occasion, need to indulge, but always

with – the key word I have learned since my operation – moderation.

Since my heart attack, I have researched healthy eating and listened to hundreds of hours of podcasts. I am by no means an expert on the subject, but I do love food and I know how important it is to us all. The overwhelming evidence points to wholefoods – the ones that have been the least-handled, manipulated or ultra-processed – being better for us. Basically, the kind of diet we all would have been eating 40 or 60 years ago. In particular, the Mediterranean diet seems to have the most health benefits – think of the many colourful ingredients we enjoy on holiday, such as fresh fish, olive oil, sun-ripened fruit, nuts and moderate (ahem) consumption of wine.

I have learned to 'eat the rainbow' – which essentially means including as many different colours of fruits and vegetables as you can in your diet – while still retaining a focus on flavour. I have used my team at the restaurant as guinea pigs for all the recipes – mainly the front of house team as they don't have the same skills as the pro team in the kitchen, and their feedback has been invaluable in creating recipes that hopefully are as foolproof as possible.

I hope this book will allow you to Eat to Your Heart's Content!

Sat Bains
Heart Attack Survivor

getting started

Umami – the fifth taste

Flavour has always been incredibly important to me, but it wasn't until I was invited to go to Japan in 2007 for an umami workshop with four other Western chefs from the UK, America and France that I really understood the importance of this fifth taste.

Umami was first identified by Japanese scientist Dr Kikunae Ikeda in 1907. Dr Ikeda found umami was made of glutamate, an amino acid that is one of the building blocks of protein. He also discovered that it was found in lots of foods, including meat, fish, fermented food and, more importantly, in mothers' breast milk, which means that as babies many of us are introduced to this rich, mouth-filling flavour very early on. Nature's very own MSG.

As a chef I found working with master chefs in Kyoto fascinating. We spent the time making dashi, preparing fish and visiting the artisans who make kombu (dried kelp) and katsuobushi (dried tuna), the building blocks of the super-savoury, high in umami stock dashi. I took so much back with me and understood that by adding ingredients rich in natural MSG to my cooking I could reduce the amount of salt I used and give my food a much cleaner flavour. I began adding anchovies to dressings, Parmesan to warm vegetables and a splash of soy here and there, which is why you will see these little hits throughout the recipes in this book.

How the chapters are organized

Eggs

Eggs, for me, are the complete wholefood. I eat them most days and love how easy they are to cook and how versatile they are. In fact, I class them as a superfood. In the past, they've had bad press. Should you eat them? How many should you eat? The truth is they are a brilliant source of protein and are both easily digestible and filling. There is nothing better than a six-egg omelette in the morning to get you going.

The recipes in this chapter are all about showcasing the many ways eggs can be cooked and encouraging you, once you've built up your cooking confidence, to go off on your own riff and start experimenting too.

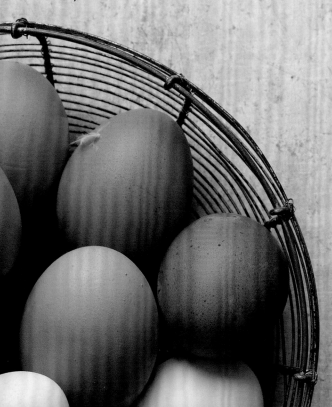

Salads

Tomato and onion, Caesar, Greek . . . I have loved salads for as long as I can remember. The diversity of textures, the fact that they can be cooling and refreshing or earthy, and that there is so much going on it is impossible to get the same ingredients in each mouthful. You will find some interesting ones in this book, which, once you are familiar with them, I hope you will be inspired to adapt to incorporate your favourite ingredients.

Vegetables

Vegetables are very versatile, but they can also be sooo boring. What I have tried to do in this chapter is showcase the diversity that the humble vegetable can bring, from the Raw cauliflower salad on page 53 and the Oven-baked carrots on page 65, to Momma Bains' chickpea curry on page 62. When Amanda and I eat at home the first thing we discuss is the vegetables we are having, as we love a table full of small pots of lots of different veggies. It really is our favourite way of eating.

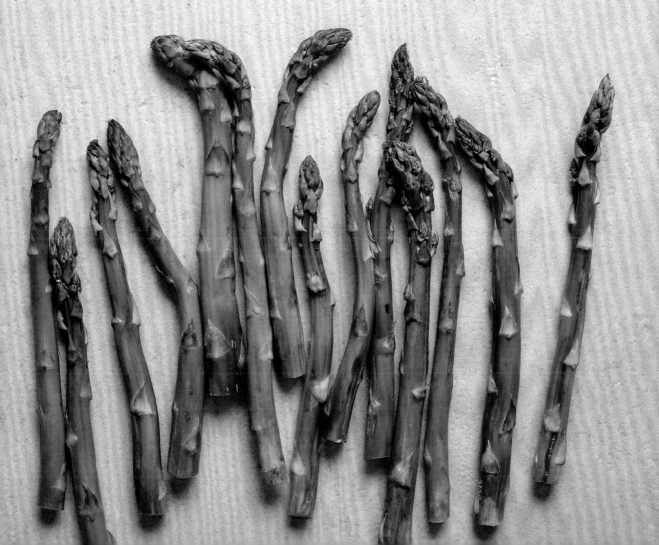

Fish

Fish, in particular oily fish, is important for heart health. Sadly, good fish can be difficult to get hold of. It's not always super fresh, but I have noticed a resurgence of local fish markets and fishmongers still providing local neighbourhoods with pristine, restaurant-quality produce. Seek out the best you can, as the results will speak for themselves. The recipes I have chosen are all easy to prepare but they do rely on quality ingredients.

Meat

I follow a high-protein diet, and meat features in it most days. As you will see in the recipes that follow, I love chicken and could eat it every day (and sometimes I do!), but I also like nothing better than a juicy 450g (1lb) medium-rare ribeye steak, although now I eat these only in moderation. I love game in season, too. It's possibly the best, healthiest meat you can eat, accompanied by a fat glass of well-aged Burgundy or Bordeaux. The following super-tasty meat dishes have all been tried and tested and don't require a professional chef's skill to cook, so I hope you will give them a go.

Smoothies, snacks and breads

I love this chapter, as these are my go-tos when I am pushed for time but still want something nutritious and filling. You can make a lot of these recipes in advanced to save even more time.

Soups, sauces, pickles and broths

If you are in a rush, these are so quick and easy to put together. Sometimes when I have trained for a long time, I don't want to eat a meal, and these just hit the spot. The dashi and bone broth are perfect meals in their own right.

Sweet things

This was a difficult one. How do you get your sweet-tooth fix when you can't eat the rubbish emulsified milk chocolate you are used to? Very difficult indeed. Especially when, like many people, I'm programmed to want something sweet after something savoury.

Growing up with a dad who owned a sweet shop, it was easy to nick a bar of chocolate here and there. After my heart attack, I told Neil about my craving for Dairy Milk. At first, I think he thought I was joking, then he got it, and laughed! Rather than deny me altogether, he allowed me either 100g (3½oz) of 70 per cent cocoa solids chocolate or two 18g (⅔oz) Freddo bars a week. Obviously I went for the Freddos, and although I'm no longer in the recovery period, I still loosely stick to the same amounts, only lapsing occasionally, as they come in packs of five or six . . .

So here I've included some alternative sweet dishes that give you your sweet hit but without all the bad stuff, like sugar and other overly processed ingredients.

Store cupboard essentials

This isn't an exhaustive list, but these are the ingredients I tend to use most frequently. I buy all my spices from my local supermarket, but wherever you get them it's best to buy them only in small quantities and to keep them in a cool, dark cupboard, as otherwise they can go stale.

Baharat
Balsamic vinegar
Chia seeds
Chilli flakes
Coriander seeds
Cumin seeds
Harissa paste (my preferred brand is Belazu)
Harissa powder
Kimchi
Miso paste
Panko breadcrumbs
Pine nuts
Pomegranate molasses
Pumpkin seeds
Preserved lemons
Ras el hanout
Rice wine vinegar
Sauerkraut
Sea salt (my preferred brand is Maldon)
Sesame seeds, both black and white
Sherry vinegar
Soy sauce
Sunflower seeds

Notes

Standard level spoon measurements are used in all recipes.

1 tablespoon = one 15ml spoon

1 teaspoon = one 5ml spoon

Eggs should be medium unless otherwise stated. The Department of Health advises that eggs should not be consumed raw. This book contains dishes made with raw or lightly cooked eggs. It is prudent for more vulnerable people such as pregnant and nursing mothers, invalids, the elderly, babies and young children to avoid uncooked or lightly cooked dishes made with eggs. Once prepared these dishes should be kept refrigerated and used promptly.

Milk should be full fat unless otherwise stated.

Fresh herbs and fresh ginger should be used unless otherwise stated. If unavailable use dried herbs as an alternative but halve the quantities stated.

Ovens should be preheated to the specific temperature – all oven temperatures are fan-assisted; if using a traditional oven, follow manufacturer's instructions for adjusting the time and the temperature.

This book includes dishes made with nuts and nut derivatives. It is advisable for those with known allergic reactions to nuts and nut derivatives and those who may be potentially vulnerable to these allergies, such as pregnant and nursing mothers, invalids, the elderly, babies and children, to avoid dishes made with nuts and nut oils. It is also prudent to check the labels of pre-prepared ingredients for the possible inclusion of nut derivatives.

Vegetarians should look for the 'V' symbol on a cheese to ensure it is made with vegetarian rennet.

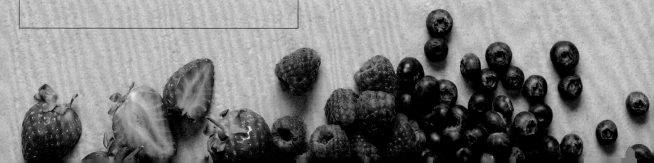

heart-healthy eating

Dr Neil Williams

Supporting Sat on writing this book has provided me with the opportunity to apply my nutrition science knowledge directly into practice – and hopefully into your kitchen, too. I hope my notes will give you a greater understanding of the power that food can have on our health.

I am often approached by patients and individuals looking for advice on the latest supplements or quick-fix diet to improve their health – perhaps to aid weight loss, or reduce their risk of cardiovascular or metabolic diseases. My response is often equivocal, because with most supplements and restrictive diets there just isn't enough evidence to give a definite answer, and our lifestyles are too complicated and nuanced for there to be a single 'cure-all'. Rather, eating recipes from this book can support a heart-healthy diet, and when combined with regular exercise and other lifestyle changes (such as stopping smoking and lowering alcohol intake) this can have proven benefits for cardiovascular health and overall wellbeing.

Throughout this book I have provided nutritional information to support the choice of ingredients for each recipe. Further context is also provided on the heart-healthy benefits of certain foods. That said, it's important to be mindful that food is more complex than individual ingredients in a recipe or the specific chemical compounds within each ingredient; rather, what is crucial is the whole complex structure and all the components of a meal. It is often too simplistic to label foods as either 'good' or 'bad'. Instead, what is known is that a well-balanced diet full of diverse and unprocessed foods will have lasting benefits to health. This book provides a fantastic collection of recipes that can support health and wellbeing, developed by one of the world's leading chefs. The recipes are centred on using a diverse range of vegetables, fruits, wholegrains, oats, nuts, pulses, lean meat, fish and shellfish, to provide something we can all enjoy.

Ecosystems such as rainforests or coral reefs are considered healthy if there is a diverse mix of animal and plant species. A similar approach can be taken with our diet – a diverse diet that includes a broad range of animal and plant-based foods will often have the greater positive health impact compared to a diet lacking diversity. Next, you will find our Top 10 heart-healthy foods. I would encourage you all to consider eating as diverse a diet as possible that includes these foods each and every week.

Dr Neil Williams is Senior Lecturer in Exercise Physiology and Nutrition at Nottingham Trent University. He has a passion for researching the role diet and nutrition play in optimising health and exercise performance and has published extensively in this area.

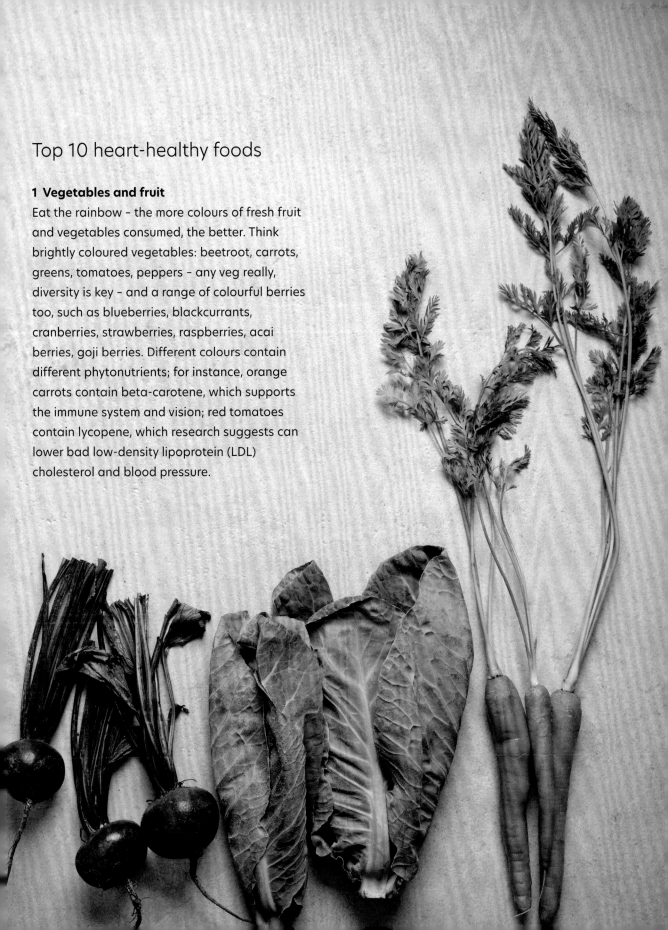

Top 10 heart-healthy foods

1 Vegetables and fruit

Eat the rainbow – the more colours of fresh fruit and vegetables consumed, the better. Think brightly coloured vegetables: beetroot, carrots, greens, tomatoes, peppers – any veg really, diversity is key – and a range of colourful berries too, such as blueberries, blackcurrants, cranberries, strawberries, raspberries, acai berries, goji berries. Different colours contain different phytonutrients; for instance, orange carrots contain beta-carotene, which supports the immune system and vision; red tomatoes contain lycopene, which research suggests can lower bad low-density lipoprotein (LDL) cholesterol and blood pressure.

- Research has shown that eating 30 different plants each week from a selection of fruits, vegetables, nuts and seeds can have a significant benefit on our gut microbiome, as well as a range of positive metabolic health outcomes

- Aim for plenty of fibrous vegetables to support heart health – think asparagus, artichoke, aubergine, okra. Fibrous vegetables can help manage cholesterol and provide a great source of prebiotic fibre, which is fuel for good gut microbes that have a range of beneficial health functions for the body. Some other prebiotic plant sources that can feed the good bugs in the gut microbiome include chicory root, dandelion root, Jerusalem artichoke, garlic, onions, leeks, asparagus, barley, oats, bananas, cocoa beans, flaxseeds and seaweed.

- Similarly, vegetables high in soluble fibre are also important for heart health; these include vegetables such as avocados and Brussels sprouts.

- Fruits high in pectin have been shown to support weight management. Pectin is a specific type of soluble fibre (a polysaccharide) found in the cell walls of fruits and vegetables. Fruits high in pectin include apples, pears, grapes, figs, strawberries and citrus fruits.

- Cruciferous vegetables are part of the Brassica genus of plants and include, but are not limited to, kale, cavolo nero, watercress, bok choy, broccoli and collard greens). They are rich in nutrients, including several carotenoids (beta-carotene, lutein, zeaxanthin); vitamins C, E and K; folate and minerals, and are a good fibre source. Research suggests the chemical compound called glucosinolate, which gives leafy greens their bitter flavour, can have an anti-inflammatory effect and support health.

- Fermented vegetables, such as sauerkraut and kimchi, can provide a great source of beneficial probiotic bacteria. Probiotics are live microorganisms, that when administered in adequate amounts, confer a health benefit to the host.

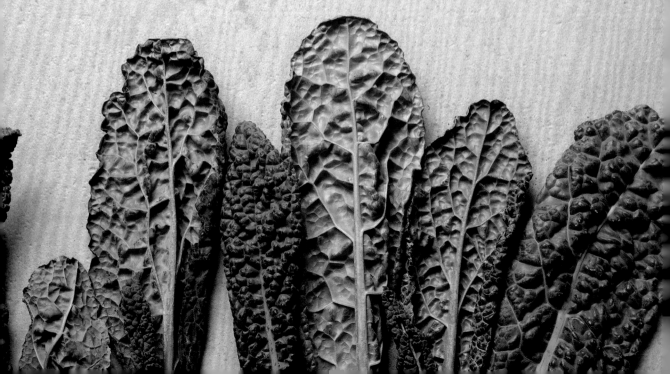

2 Oats and barley

Oats and barley are grains rich in a type of fibre called beta-glucan. When you eat beta-glucan it forms a gel that binds to cholesterol-rich bile acids in the gut. This helps limit the amount of cholesterol that is absorbed from the gut into your blood. Several studies now show that eating 3g (0.1oz) of beta-glucan a day as part of a healthy diet and lifestyle can lower cholesterol.

3 Beans and pulses

Beans are especially rich in soluble fibre. They also take a while for the body to digest, meaning you feel full for longer after a meal, therefore reducing the chance of overeating, which leads to weight gain – a key risk factor for cardiovascular disease. Black beans and butter (lima) beans contain some of the highest soluble-fibre content, but consider increasing your dietary intake of all types of beans and pulses, as this will increase the fibre content of a meal – something Western diets are typically lacking in.

4 Extra virgin olive oil

Extra virgin olive oil is loaded with monounsaturated fatty acids (MUFAs), types of fatty acids that have been linked to several health benefits. Specifically, research suggests that MUFAs can benefit heart health and may even protect against heart disease by reducing inflammation and bad cholesterol while also increasing good cholesterol.

5 Nuts and seeds

Nuts are a good source of unsaturated fats and are lower in saturated fats, both of which can help to keep your cholesterol in check. They contain fibre, which can help block some cholesterol being absorbed into the bloodstream from the gut, as well as protein, vitamin E, magnesium, potassium, natural plant sterols and other plant nutrients that can support health. Their high protein and fibre content help to keep you full, so you're less likely to snack on other things, too. Aim for around 30g (1oz) of nuts a day; all fresh nuts count, so again, choose a variety that includes hazelnuts, almonds, macadamia nuts, Brazil nuts, cashew nuts, pistachios, walnuts, peanuts and pecans. Aim to eat them in place of another snack or include them as part of a meal. Where possible, go for nuts with their skins still intact.

Again, including a variety of seeds in the diet is great. A particular star is flaxseed, which has a high omega-3 and fibre content and can also be considered a prebiotic. Sunflower seeds are also a good option.

6 Soya bean/soya products

There is some encouraging evidence that eating soya-based products (those especially high in a soya bean protein called beta-conglycinin) can help lower LDL cholesterol.

7 Oily fish

Eating oily fish, such as salmon, sardines or mackerel, two or three times a week can lower LDL cholesterol; the high levels of omega-3 polyunsaturated fatty acids they offer can help reduce triglycerides in the bloodstream and protect the heart by helping prevent the onset of abnormal heart rhythms.

8 Shellfish

Shellfish are high in protein and low in fat. The levels of protein and iron in mussels can rival those found in any red meat on a menu. Protein and iron are fundamental to health, providing the body's building blocks and delivering oxygen to cells. Mussels and clams are also packed full of omega-3 polyunsaturated fatty acids, zinc and vitamin B12. Crab also has a good nutrient content and is a lean protein source.

9 Lean meat

White meat, such as turkey and chicken, is lower in saturated fat than red meat and provides an excellent source of protein and essential amino acids, which are the building blocks of our cells and tissues in our body.

There is a lot of contention regarding the negative health effects of red meat intake and heart disease. Some studies demonstrate an increased risk when consuming unprocessed and processed red meat, while a few show an increased risk for only processed meat, and others report no significant association at all. So where does that leave us? Well, first we must keep in mind that observational studies cannot prove cause and effect, they can only demonstrate that meat eaters are either more or less likely to get a disease. It could be that meat consumption is just a marker of unhealthy lifestyle behaviours, but not a sole effect of red meat itself. Further, our diets should not be restrictive, rather, we should just consider that moderate unprocessed red meat intake can form part of a diverse diet.

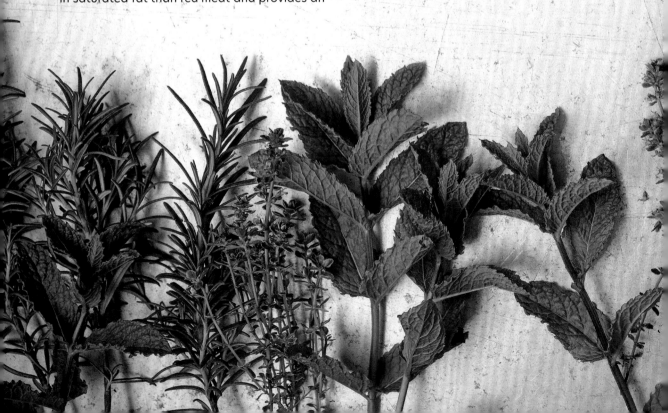

So when it comes to meat selection, we should make sure we are getting the best cut of meat for the most benefits and nutrients. A heart-healthy diet can also include a moderate intake of lean cuts of red meat, such as venison and lamb. For a well-balanced diet, nothing should really be off the menu. Diversity is key to health, but it's important to be mindful that this also means moderation of some components.

10 Spices and herbs

There is now ample evidence that spices and herbs possess antioxidant, anti-inflammatory, antitumorigenic (counteracting the formation of tumours), anticarcinogenic and glucose- and cholesterol-lowering properties, as well as having a positive impact on cognition and mood. These little nutrient powerhouses should be included as part of a diverse diet. Not only will they elevate the taste of any meal, but adding them to most, if not all, meals provides ample opportunity to ingest the health-benefiting compounds found in spices and herbs to support health.

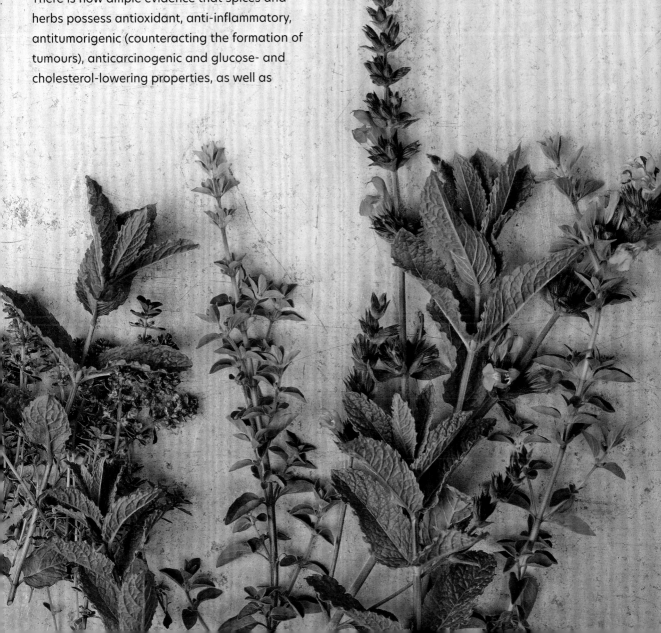

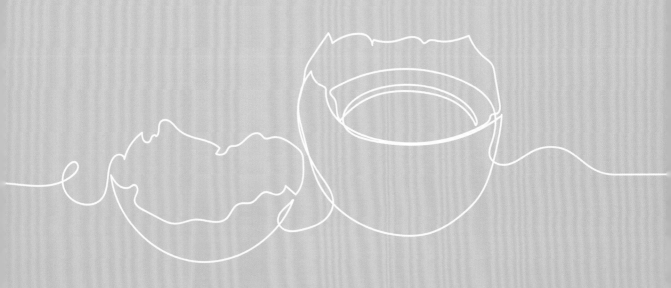

1

eggs

'Sat-Shuka' baked eggs with stewed leeks and chilli

I have this a couple of times a month as a brunch, and I find that the more you make it, the more confident you become, then you can start experimenting with switching in different vegetables and spices. Amanda's favourite vegetable is leek and her best ever dish is a French classic called étuvée of leeks, which is basically braised leeks that are sliced very thinly and cooked with a splash of water and a knob of butter in a pan with a lid on, so this dish was inspired by that. You can add kale, pak choi or any other greens you like to replace the spinach, if you prefer.

Nutrition notes

Like other members of the onion family, leeks are packed with nutrients and contain high amounts of flavonoid antioxidants, minerals and vitamins. They are a particularly good source of kaempferol, a polyphenol antioxidant that, in some laboratory studies, has been shown to support our cardiovascular system by protecting the lining of our blood vessels. The elongated stem of the leek is also an excellent source of soluble and insoluble fibre, making this vegetable a great choice to improve gut health and support the community of good bugs in our guts.

Equipment | 18cm x 8cm (7in x 3in) casserole pot with a lid

1   Pour the olive oil and butter into the casserole pot and place on a medium heat. Add the leeks and the cumin seeds and season with salt and pepper, then cover with the lid and cook until the leeks are soft, 5–7 minutes.

2   Remove the lid and add the spinach, then stir over the heat until wilted. Make a well in the mix and gently drop in the eggs one by one. Replace the lid and cook for 3–5 minutes or until the eggs are gently cooked – you want to make sure these are soft-poached.

3   Remove the lid and season the eggs with salt and pepper and sprinkle over the chilli flakes.

Serves 2

50ml (2fl oz) extra virgin olive oil
50g (2oz) butter
200g (7oz) leeks, finely sliced, washed and drained
1 teaspoon toasted cumin seeds
100g (3½oz) baby spinach, washed
4 large organic eggs, cracked individually into small bowls or cups
½ teaspoon chilli flakes
Flaked sea salt and freshly ground black pepper, to taste

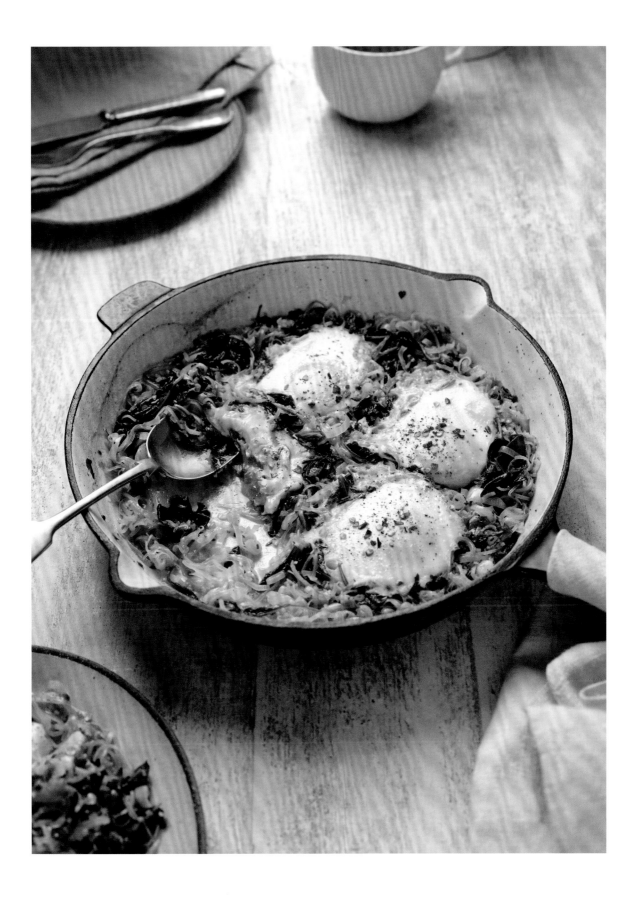

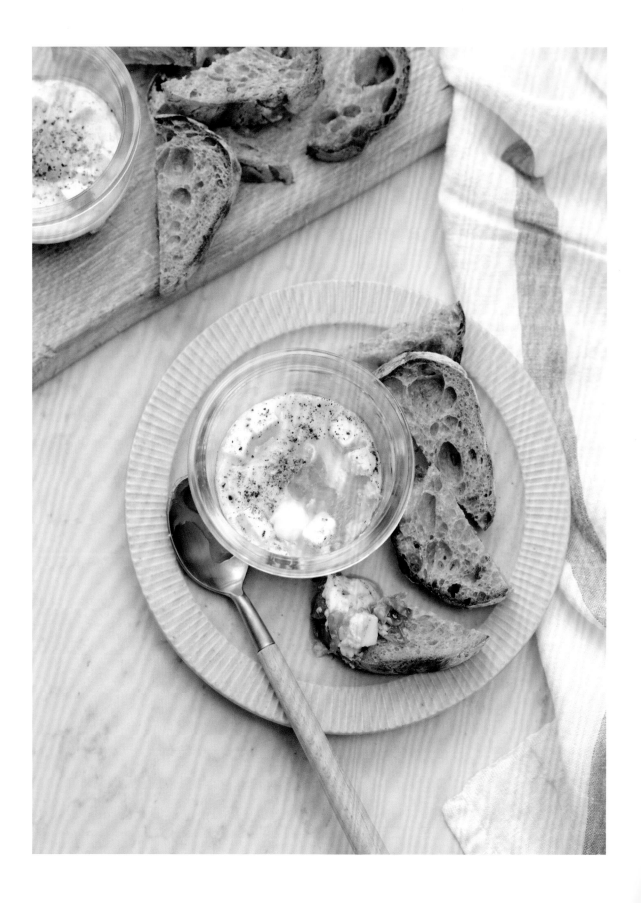

Coddled eggs with caramelized onions and feta

Coddled eggs go back centuries. There is no record of when egg coddlers were invented or who was the first to manufacture them, but they started to become popular in Europe in the late nineteenth century. The first known Worcester coddlers were made at Grainger's China Works in the 1880s, and were made of earthenware, which was fired at a very high temperature. With evolution we can now use glass and earthenware pots as well as ceramics, and we can even coddle eggs in their shells, using a Japanese technique called onsen tamago, where eggs are cooked in hot-water springs at a perfect 62-65°C (144-149°F) - their natural temperature.

Equipment | 4 ovenproof glass or ceramic ramekins

1   In a saucepan heat some olive oil over a medium heat, then add the onions and cook gently to slowly caramelize them. This will take 30-40 minutes, so be patient - but it is worth it.

2   Preheat the oven to 160°C/350°F. Brush the ramekins with the melted butter and line a tray that can fit the 4 ramekins in with some kitchen towel.

3   Divide the onion mix equally between the buttered ramekin dishes. Gently crack an egg into each ramekin and season with salt and pepper. Add the diced feta cheese and cover each pot with ovenproof clingfilm. Place these on a deep tray and add some hot water to create a water bath. Place in the oven and cook for 10-15 minutes or until there is a slight wobble.

4   Remove the clingfilm and leave to rest for a few minutes. Now enjoy.

Sat's tip: The kitchen towel in step 3 allows the ramekins to sit snugly in the tray so they don't move when you are carrying them to the oven.

Serves 2

Olive oil, for frying
2 sweet white onions, very
    thinly sliced
Melted butter, for
    brushing the ramekins
4 super-fresh eggs
50g (2oz) feta cheese,
    diced
Flaked sea salt and
    freshly ground black
    pepper, to taste

Fried eggs in lots of olive oil and chilli (Egg Banjo)

I was introduced to this dish by my old mentor Mick Murphy in the early 1990s. He had just come back from Spain and this is the dish he gave me on first meeting him; I have tweaked it a little by adding chilli flakes. The reason it was called a Banjo is something I've learned only recently. The egg was always cooked with a runny yolk, so when you bit into your cob/sandwich or bap, the yolk would dribble down your shirt while you tried to clean up the mess and imitated playing a banjo ... ha ha ha! (This new information is courtesy of Gerald from Geralds Bar in Melbourne, Australia, in his recently released book.)

Nutrition notes

Extra virgin olive oil is loaded with monounsaturated fatty acids (MUFAs), a type of healthy fat that has been linked to several health benefits. Research suggests that, specifically when consumed as part of a diverse Mediterranean diet, MUFAs can benefit heart health and may even protect against heart disease by reducing inflammation and bad cholesterol, while increasing good cholesterol.

Serves 2

100ml (3½fl oz) olive oil
2 garlic cloves, crushed
    with skin on
4 large organic eggs
Pinch of dried chilli flakes
Flaked sea salt and
    freshly ground black
    pepper, to taste

1   Heat the olive oil in a non-stick frying pan on a medium heat. Add the garlic and let it infuse the oil.

2   One at a time, crack the eggs into a bowl and gently slide into the hot oil. Scatter over the chilli flakes followed by a sprinkling of salt and pepper. Gently cook the eggs to your liking until all four are cooked and serve straightaway in a toasted sandwich or sourdough cob.

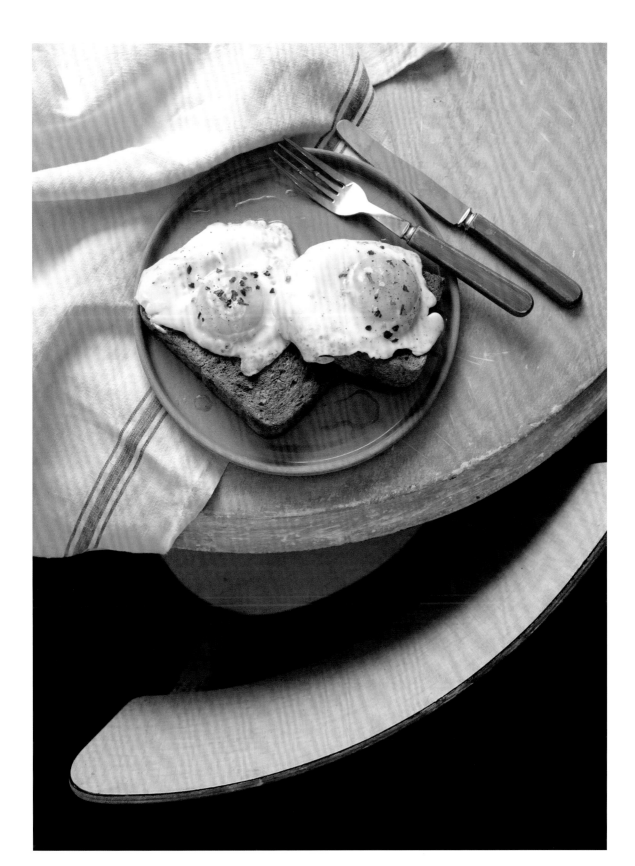

Blended omelette with spinach and feta

This has got to be one of the easiest and simplest recipes in this book. If you're short on time or just want something delicious quickly, this is for you.

Nutrition notes

Eggs are crammed full of nutrients and protein. The combination of eggs and feta cheese in this omelette means it is a simple protein-packed meal. Gram for gram, both eggs and feta provide a great source of protein, which helps us to feel satiated (full) after eating and means we are less likely to snack on unhealthy food options. Further, the combination of these protein sources provides the essential amino acids that our bodies require to build muscle, meaning this recipe is a speedy post-exercise meal option.

Equipment | Blender

1   Preheat your grill.

2   Place the eggs and spinach into a blender and blend on full for 30 seconds. Add the feta and pulse a few times just until the cheese has broken down. Season with a pinch each of salt and pepper.

3   Place a non-stick frying pan on a medium heat and drizzle in a little olive oil. Add the omelette mix and gently cook, using a spatula to keep the mix moving until it has semi-set.

4   Place under the grill and cook the top of the omelette until set and browned to your liking.

Serves 2

4 large organic eggs
200g (7oz) baby spinach
100g (3½oz) feta cheese, roughly broken up
Flaked sea salt and freshly ground white pepper, to taste
Extra virgin olive oil, for frying

Chorizo eggs with coriander

Probably my all-time favourite breakfast – you may have noticed I love eggs? The best part of this dish is the release of the delicious orange-paprika, chilli-infused oil that is released from frying the chorizo sausages; this adds a beautiful golden hue to the eggs. If you can get it, go for piquant chorizo, as it is slightly spicier. I serve this with smashed avocado: a perfect breakfast.

Nutrition notes

Eggs are such a great nutritional choice and should form a staple of any diverse diet. Coriander includes some important compounds that when eaten as part of a balanced diet, may support health. Albeit primarily from rodent studies, the antioxidant compounds of terpinene, quercetin and tocopherols, found in coriander, may have immune-boosting, anticancer and neuroprotective effects. Also, some rodent models offer promising evidence that coriander may lower the heart disease risk factor of high blood pressure, as well as LDL-cholesterol.

Equipment | Blender

1   Start by making the coriander salt. Place the coriander seeds and cinnamon bark in a blender and pulse for around 30 seconds. Add the salt and pulse once or twice to combine. Place in an airtight container and store in the fridge until needed.

2   Heat the olive oil in a non-stick pan over a medium heat, then add the chorizo. Fry until the chorizo is starting to caramelize, which will take around 10 minutes. At this point the chorizo will start releasing its own oils, and some of this can be drained off before adding the eggs.

3   Add the eggs to the pan and gently cook for around 5 minutes or until the eggs are starting to set. Season with the coriander salt and pepper, and sprinkle with some fresh coriander to serve.

Sat's tip: This recipe will make more coriander salt than needed, but it can be used throughout the recipes in this book. The salt is best used within 3–6 months, it can't spoil in effect, but the aroma can diminish

Serves 2

25ml (1fl oz) extra virgin
    olive oil
50g (2oz) chorizo, diced
4 large organic eggs
Freshly ground black
    pepper, to taste
Freshly chopped
    coriander, to serve

For the coriander salt
25g (1oz) toasted
    coriander seeds
10g (¼oz) toasted
    cinnamon bark
200g (7oz) flaked sea salt

Leftover vegetable 'Spanish tortilla'

I use this method a lot if I have cooked lots of vegetables and have them leftover – there is nothing better than throwing a few eggs into a frying pan with all your leftovers, and within 10 or 15 minutes having a substantial meal and having saved on waste, time and effort but not compromised on flavour. I like to eat mine with a side of kimchi.

Serves 2

250g (9oz) any leftover
   cooked vegetables,
   coarsely chopped
6 large organic eggs
1 teaspoon chilli flakes
30ml (1fl oz) olive oil
Flaked sea salt and freshly
   ground black pepper, to
   taste

1   In a large mixing bowl add the chopped vegetables, crack in the eggs and mix. Add the chilli flakes, salt and pepper and mix again.

2   Add the olive oil to the pan on a medium heat and wait until it is hot, then gently add the egg mix. Using a spatula, move the mix around slowly to make sure it cooks evenly, shaking the pan every now and then to make sure the tortilla is free.

3   Now get a large dinner plate and place it on top of the pan, then flip the pan using oven gloves to turn out the tortilla onto the plate. It should be golden brown. Slide the tortilla back into the pan to carry on cooking the bottom, which was the top!

4   When cooked, turn off the heat and let the tortilla cool in the pan. Once cool, slide onto a chopping board, slice and serve.

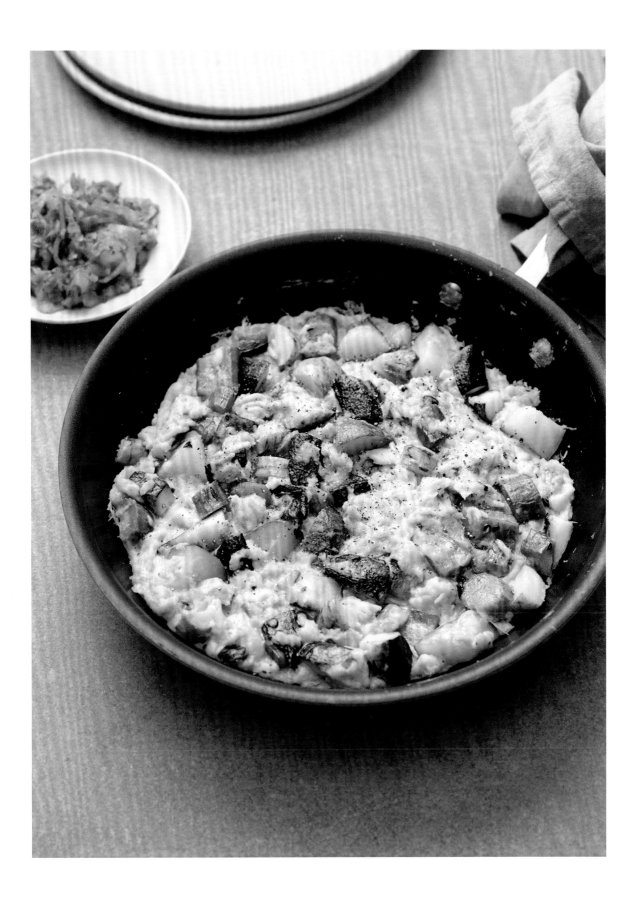

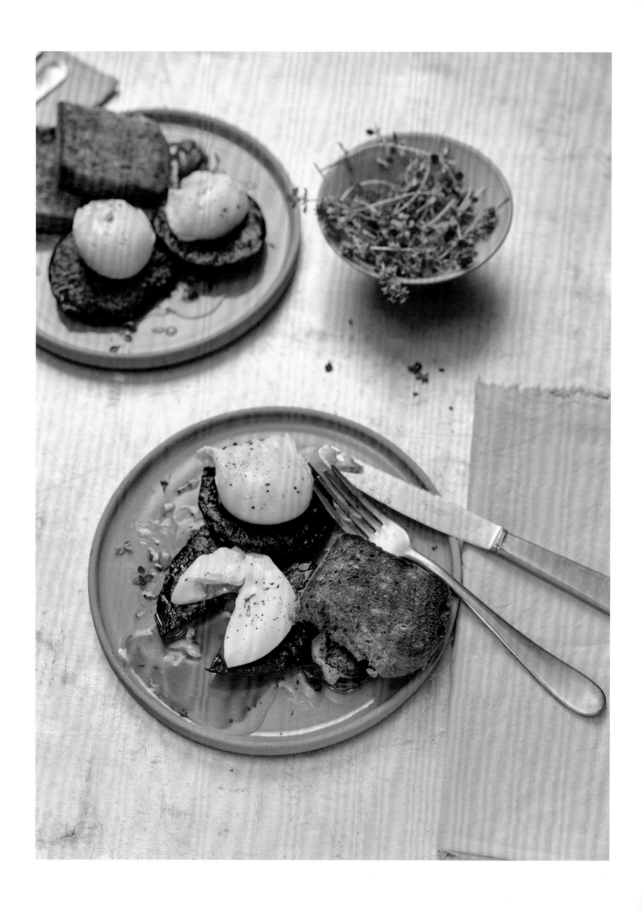

Pot-roast mushrooms with poached eggs and thyme

The mushrooms in this dish have a meat-like texture. I prefer my eggs soft poached so that when cooked they mix with the pan juices and create a beautiful sauce. I sometimes add any leftover Four-bean chilli (see page 140) to the mushrooms and top with the poached eggs for a more substantial meal.

Nutrition notes

Eggs used to get a bad rap because of their high cholesterol content and suggestions they would raise blood cholesterol. This fact originated from what is now considered an outdated understanding; updated evidence shows that eggs do not have a significant effect on blood cholesterol. The truth is, eggs are cracking! They are a natural source of high-quality protein as well as vitamin B2 (also known as riboflavin), which is essential for the growth, development and function of cells in the body. Eggs are also rich in selenium, which is an antioxidant beneficial for our immune system, thyroid function and mental health.

Equipment | 18cm x 8cm (7in x 3in) casserole pot with a lid

1   Preheat the oven to 160°C/350°F.

2   Heat the olive oil in the casserole pot on a high heat. Add the mushrooms topside down and cook for 3 minutes or until golden brown. Add the butter and turn down the heat. Turn over and gently cook the mushrooms for a further few minutes until caramelized.

3   Add the garlic and thyme, place the lid on the pot, transfer to the oven and cook for 20 minutes.

4   About 5 minutes before the mushrooms come out of the oven, poach your eggs in a pan of salted simmering water.

5   Remove the mushrooms from the oven and leave to cool for a few minutes. Transfer to a plate and place the poached eggs on top. Spoon over the juices from the mushrooms and serve.

Serves 2

75ml (3fl oz) extra virgin olive oil
4 large portobello mushrooms, cleaned and stalks removed
25g (1oz) salted butter
2 garlic cloves, crushed
10 sprigs of thyme
4 large organic eggs
Flaked sea salt and freshly ground black pepper, to taste

Shiitake mushrooms with beluga lentils and fried eggs

A fricassee of mushrooms is one of the most evocative, delicious things I can imagine: earthy notes, meaty mushrooms – and who doesn't love a fried egg? The beluga lentils add a great texture to the dish, and garlic and thyme are just meant for each other. You can try other mushrooms here, if you like.

Nutrition notes

This recipe is crammed full of lovely flavoured nutritional goodness. Shiitake mushrooms increase our all-important daily vegetable intake here, and they contain the heart-healthy soluble fibre beta-glucan (see also page 174), which can reduce insulin resistance, lower cholesterol and support body weight and heart health. Mushrooms are also high in potassium, which is important for heart function. Combining these great mushrooms with lentils means this recipe is very high in fibre, supporting overall heart and gut health.

Equipment | Large non-stick frying pan with a lid

1   Cut the mushrooms into nice even slices, about 2cm (¾in), but still keeping them large enough to create texture. Add the olive oil to the pan until it gets nice and hot, then add the mushrooms. Turn up the heat and sauté for several minutes until lovely and toasted, then turn the heat down a little and heat the butter until it melts and bubbles. Add the garlic, shallots and thyme and stir well for a few moments, then add the beluga lentils and stir to coat.

2   Make 2 wells in the mixture and crack an egg into each one. Pop the lid on and cook for 4–5 minutes or until the eggs are beautifully cooked. Season with salt and pepper and serve.

Serves 1

200g (7oz) shiitake mushrooms, wiped clean
50ml (1¾fl oz) olive oil
40g (1½oz) salted butter
3 garlic cloves, crushed
2 shallots, finely sliced
2 sprigs of thyme
1 x 100g (3½oz) pouch of precooked beluga lentils
2 large organic eggs, cracked into 2 small bowls
Flaked sea salt and freshly ground black pepper, to taste

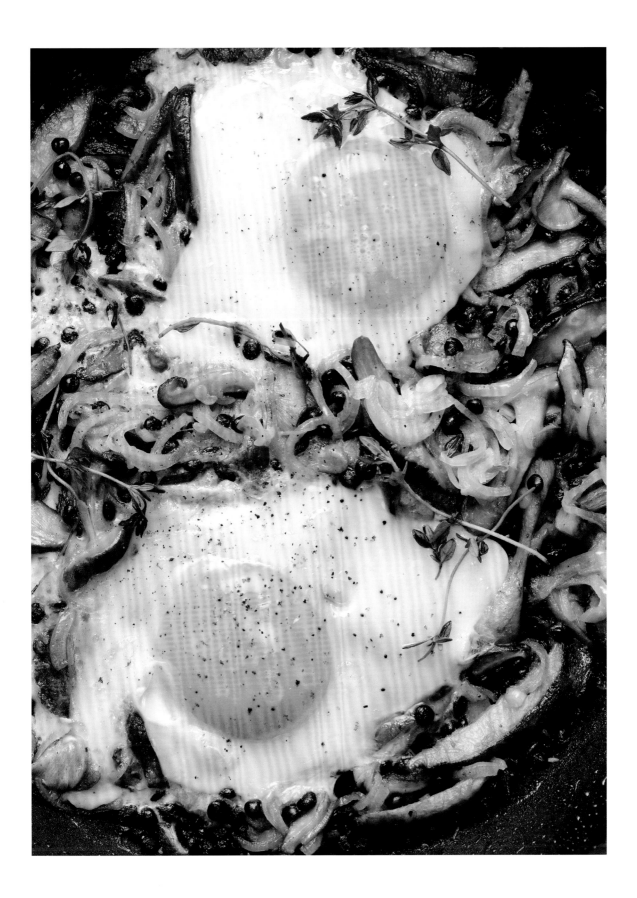

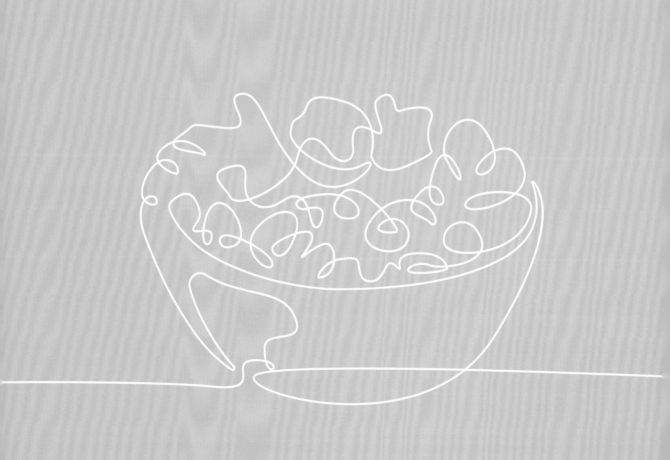

2

salads

Crudités

What a brilliant way to get loads of crunchy, ice-cold, healthy vegetables into you! Amanda and I have this on a Sunday afternoon, with hummus and a broad bean purée. The secret is to prepare all the vegetables in advance and let them chill for at least 2 hours – it makes for a perfect hot summer's day with a nice glass of chilled wine.

Nutrition notes

This is a simple way to get the many benefits of consuming fresh vegetables in a variety of colours, tastes and textures. Vegetables are packed with phytochemicals, such as polyphenols, glucosinolates and carotenoids. However, some cooking methods – think boiling the life out of green vegetables – can reduce the concentration of phytochemicals, especially polyphenols. This recipe contains also raw chicory, which is one of the best sources of prebiotic fibres (inulin and fructooligosaccharides), helping to feed the good bacteria in the gut and resulting in a wide range of health benefits.

Serves 2

2 long red peppers
1 red chicory
1 yellow chicory
8 radishes
1 Granny Smith apple
1 medium carrot
16 sugar snap peas
1 red onion
½ medium cucumber
1 baby gem lettuce
Flaked sea salt, to taste

1   Top and tail the long red peppers, remove the seeds and cut into strips. Remove the bottom of the chicory stems and pull away the leaves, and place in a bowl of ice-cold water for 10 minutes. Cut the radishes in half, wash in cold water and drain on kitchen towel. Cut the apple into 8 wedges and remove the core, then season with a pinch of salt. Peel the carrot, remove the top and bottom, cut in half widthways, then cut into 8 batons per piece. Top and tail the sugar snap peas. Peel the red onion and cut into 16 wedges. Peel the cucumber, cut in half, remove the seeds and cut into 8 lengthways.

2   Remove the stem of the baby gem lettuce, pull apart the leaves and wash in ice-cold water.

3   Arrange on a platter and serve alongside your preferred dip.

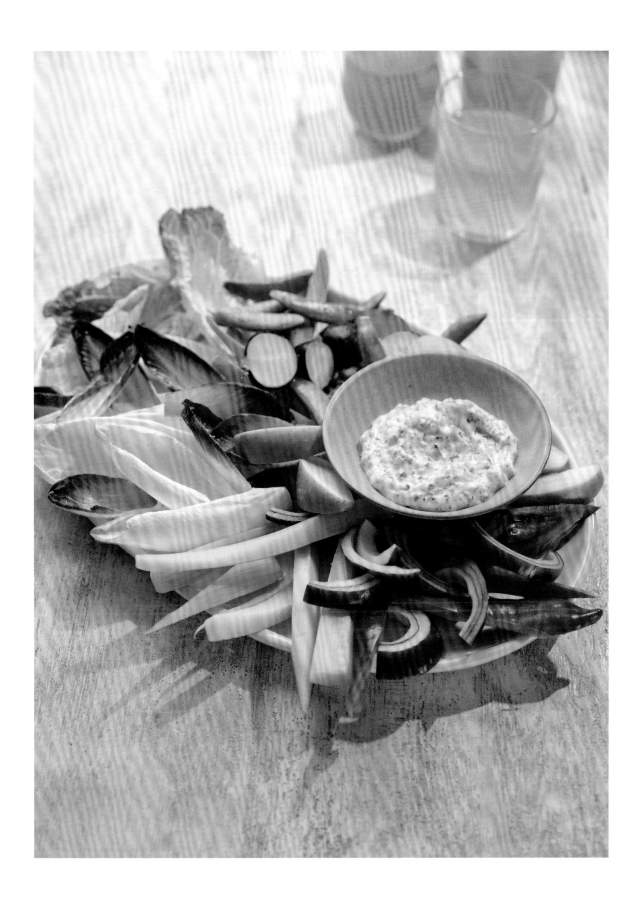

My Greek salad

Me and Amanda love the Greek isles for our holidays in summer. I always ask for a big Greek salad wherever I go, but sometimes there are no onions, sometimes no olives, so I have made my favourite version of all time with everything I want in it. The secret of this salad is to keep it chunky so you can get your fork in, with loads of variety on the end of it.

🫁 **Nutrition notes**

Diversity is key to a healthy diet, and this Greek salad has great nutritional diversity thanks to a broad combination of ingredients. A Greek salad is a good example of eating the rainbow, with red tomatoes (getting their lovely red flesh from the healthy carotenoid compound called lycopene), green cucumber (thanks to chlorophyll), red onions (getting their lovely purple colour from the antioxidant compounds of anthocyanins and flavonoids), and green olives (which are high in polyphenols as well as a heart-healthy mono-unsaturated fatty acid called oleic acid). The combination of these fantastic vegetables served with a healthy dose of extra virgin olive oil, and it's no wonder the Mediterranean is consistently associated with lower cardiovascular disease risk and mortality.

Serves 2

1. Place all the ingredients into a bowl and gently combine. Season with salt and pepper and leave for 30 minutes before serving.

2 ripe plum tomatoes, cut into 8 wedges each

½ medium cucumber, peeled, deseeded and cut into 2cm (¾in) chunks

1 small red onion, chopped into 2-3cm (¾-1¼in) pieces

100g (3½oz) barrel-aged feta cheese, cut into 3cm (1¼in) dice

10g (¼oz) basil leaves, torn

1 teaspoon tiny capers

10 pitted big green olives, cut in half

5g fresh oregano, finely sliced

1 tablespoon extra virgin olive oil

1 teaspoon white wine vinegar

Flaked sea salt and freshly ground black pepper, to taste

My warm Asian spinach

The simplicity of this dish is unbelievable for the payoff in flavour. You can also cook broccoli, kale and most green veg in the same style.

Spinach is loaded with healthy nutrients and high in insoluble fibre, which improves digestion, keeping you regular and looking after your gut. Spinach is very high in vitamin K, which supports blood clotting, and also contains antioxidants, which fight oxidative stress and help reduce the damage it causes. One study found that daily consumption of spinach helped to prevent oxidative damage and although this was a small-scale study in humans, it is supported by other animal studies.

Serves 2

1   Mix all the ingredients together for the dressing in a large bowl and set aside.

2   Cook the spinach in a large pan with the olive oil until wilted. When cooked, place straight in the bowl with the dressing. Mix well and place into a serving bowl.

400g (14oz) baby spinach, washed and drained
1 teaspoon extra virgin olive oil

For the dressing
1 teaspoon grated ginger
1 teaspoon grated garlic
1 teaspoon soy sauce
1 tablespoon extra virgin olive oil
½ teaspoon dried chilli flakes

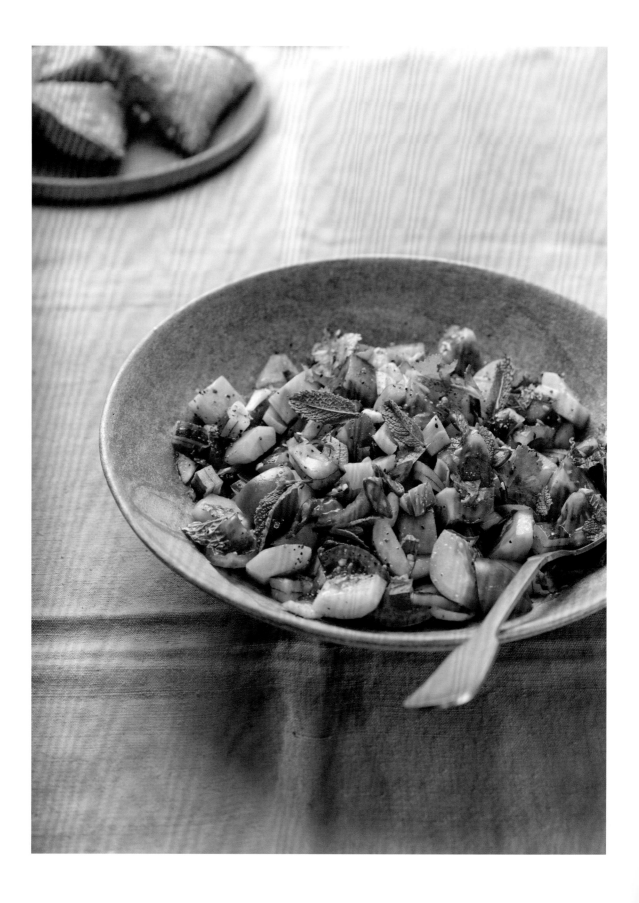

My Punjabi salad

Growing up in a Punjabi household, salad was a strange thing. We used to serve it in the middle of the table and it always consisted of cucumber, tomato and white Spanish onion, all either sliced thick or chopped thick, always sprinkled with fine table salt and white ground pepper. I think this is where my love of salads was born; I loved the fizz in the nose from the extra-hot Spanish onion and the cooling effect of the cucumber, the sweetness from the tomato and the salt and pepper. Here I have reinvented my childhood salad; adding paneer gives it a lovely texture, while a dash of chilli brings heat. It is one of the easiest salads to prepare.

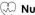 **Nutrition notes**

Yet another example of a delicious salad full of a diverse range of vegetables and herbs. Different-coloured fruit, vegetables, herbs and spices all contain different nutrients and bioactive compounds, including, amongst others, phytochemicals (phenolics, flavonoids and carotenoids), vitamins (vitamin C, folate and provitamin A), minerals (potassium, calcium and magnesium) and fibres. Therefore, the wider the variety of fruit, vegetables, herbs and spices we eat, the increased likelihood there is that we are going to be ingesting suitable amounts of these health-benefiting nutrients and compounds.

1   Place all the ingredients into a large bowl and mix well.

2   Scatter the reserved herbs at the end and serve.

Serves 2

2 ripe plum tomatoes, cut into 8 wedges each

½ medium cucumber, peeled, deseeded and cut into 2cm (¾in) chunks

1 small red onion cut into 2cm (¾in) dice

1 red chilli, deseeded and finely sliced (add the seeds if you like it a bit spicier)

10g (¼oz) coriander leaves, finely sliced (save half to finish)

10g (¼oz) mint leaves, finely sliced (save half to finish)

1 tablespoon extra virgin olive oil

Flaked sea salt and freshly ground black pepper, to taste

My spinach Caesar salad

Caesar salad? Who doesn't love it, I also love baby spinach in salads, so here it is – all the salad components but with super-healthy spinach instead of lettuce. I have this as a side with chicken, my lamb chops and, obviously, a good steak.

Nutrition notes

Anchovies are a little fish with a big nutritional value. They are considered an oily fish alongside salmon, mackerel and sardines and have a high heart-healthy content of omega-3 polyunsaturated fatty acids known as DHA and EPA. One study showed that a daily intake of 566mg of DHA and EPA combined could lower the risk of death from heart disease. You can easily obtain that amount of omega-3s from a 45g (2oz) tin of anchovies.

1 Place all the ingredients except the spinach and salt into a large bowl. Whisk until fully combined and emulsified.

2 Throw in your baby spinach and gently toss in the mixture to coat. Season with a little salt if needed.

Serves 2

75g (3oz) Parmesan, grated
Zest and juice of 1 lemon
1 garlic clove, grated
1 egg yolk
15g (½oz) anchovies, chopped (I use Ortiz)
50ml (2fl oz) extra virgin olive oil
200g (7oz) pre-washed baby spinach
Flaked sea salt, to taste

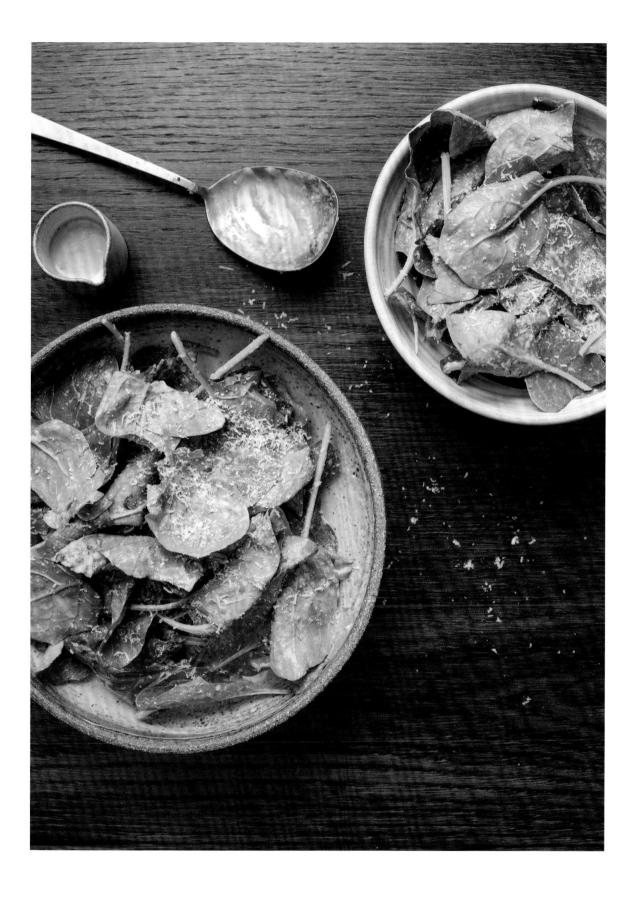

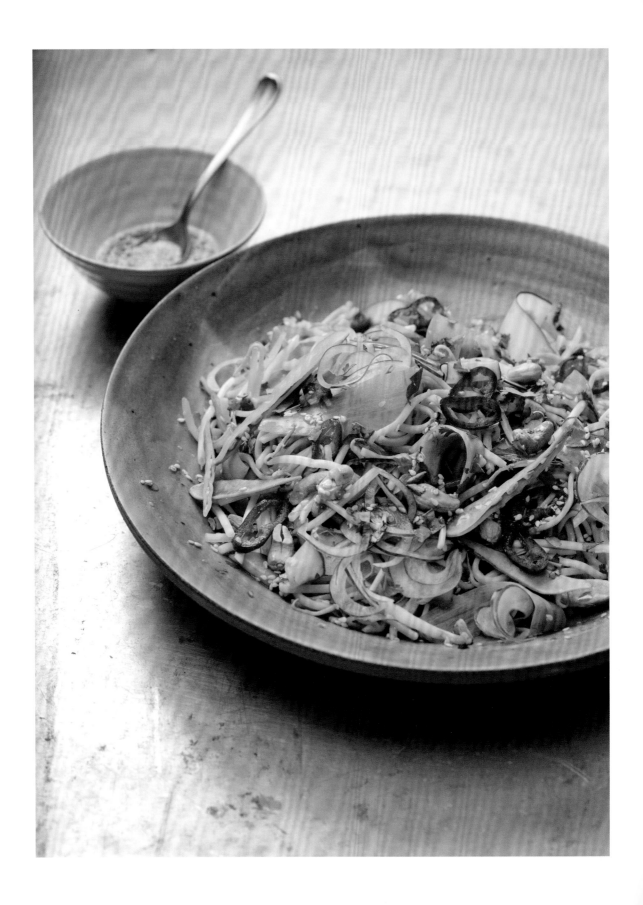

Noodle and shaved vegetable salad

Amanda loves this salad and we have it with the Cod baked in parchment (page 95). Super light, it deceptively looks like a lot but surprisingly, once dressed and having been left to marinate for a few minutes, it reduces in size because the dressing slowly breaks down the fresh vegetables. You could easily polish off two portions on your own - or I could anyway... ha ha!

The nam pla adds a funkiness to this salad, but once you get over the smell, you will, like me, become addicted.

Nutrition notes

Mangetout are essentially a type of pea, so these come from the legume family. The name in French means 'eat all', and by doing just that we can get a high fibre and vitamin C intake with this little pea. Vitamin C contributes to many functions in our body, including maintaining healthy blood vessels, bones and cartilage. Vitamin C also plays an important role in supporting our immune system, and there is some evidence that when exposed to physical stress (such as high exercise training load), vitamin C supplementation may reduce the incidence of colds.

Equipment | A mandoline would be perfect to get the veg wafer thin, if not, use a very sharp knife.

1   In a large bowl, mix all of the salad ingredients together. In a separate bowl, combine all the dressing ingredients.

2   Tip the salad ingredients into the dressing, toss to combine and leave to marinate for 10 minutes before serving.

Serves 2

1 medium carrot, peeled and finely sliced
1 red onion, finely sliced
½ medium cucumber, peeled, deseeded and finely sliced
½ courgette, finely sliced
50g (2oz) mangetout, finely sliced
100g (3½oz) beansprouts, cut in half
½ teaspoon toasted white sesame seeds
10g (¼oz) fresh coriander, finely chopped
1 x 250g (9oz) pack of cooked egg noodles

For the dressing
2 teaspoons soy sauce
1 teaspoon sesame oil
1 teaspoon nam pla
1 teaspoon chilli flakes
1 teaspoon rice wine vinegar
100ml (3½fl oz) extra virgin olive oil

Triple-layered tomato, onion, fennel and basil salad

This is probably one of my favourite salads of all time, I like it with a juicy ribeye, roast chicken or just on its own, super chilled and straight from the fridge on a hot summer's day. You can also bring it up to room temperature, allowing all the flavours to meld. One of the best parts of this dish is the juices it leaves at the bottom of the plate – get some sourdough and soak it all up.

Nutrition notes

Tomatoes are a great, ripe fruit providing an excellent source of essential nutrients. Tomatoes get their bright red pigment from a phytonutrient carotenoid called lycopene, but the name isn't as important as what they can do. Lycopene-containing foods have been shown to lower bad (LDL) cholesterol and blood pressure, both of which are really important to help maintain heart health. Reducing LDL cholesterol reduces the risk of atherosclerosis (plaque build-up in the arteries), and aids in reducing blood pressure. Lower blood pressure significantly lowers the risk of heart attack and stroke. The raw onion in this salad is a fantastic source of inulin and fructooligosaccharides, which are prebiotics. Prebiotics feed the good bugs in your gut, which can improve overall gut health and immunity.

1 Arrange one-third of the sliced tomatoes on a large, flat plate. Season with salt and pepper.

2 Mix together the vinaigrette ingredients in a small bowl or jug.

3 Add half of the fennel and onion to the tomatoes, and drizzle over 1 tablespoon of the vinaigrette. Repeat this process again, starting with another layer of tomatoes, then finish with a layer of the remaining tomatoes. Leave for 1 hour before serving.

Serves 2

6 super-ripe plum tomatoes, sliced as thinly as possible

1 medium red onion, sliced as thinly as possible

1 fennel bulb, sliced as thinly as possible

25g (1oz) fresh basil leaves, torn at the last minute

Flaked sea salt and freshly ground black pepper, to taste

For the vinaigrette

100ml (3½fl oz) extra virgin olive oil

25ml (1fl oz) sherry vinegar

20ml (½fl oz) soy sauce

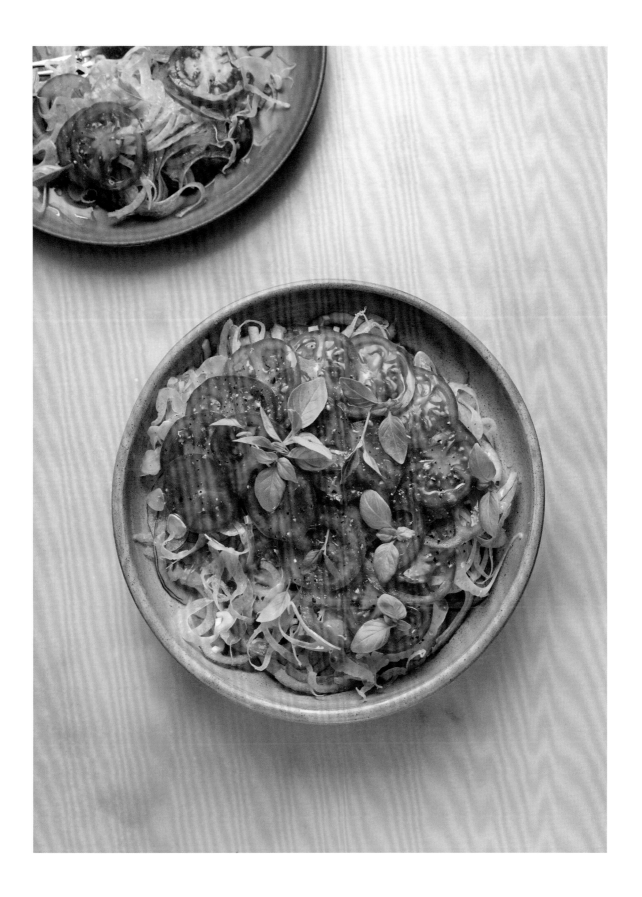

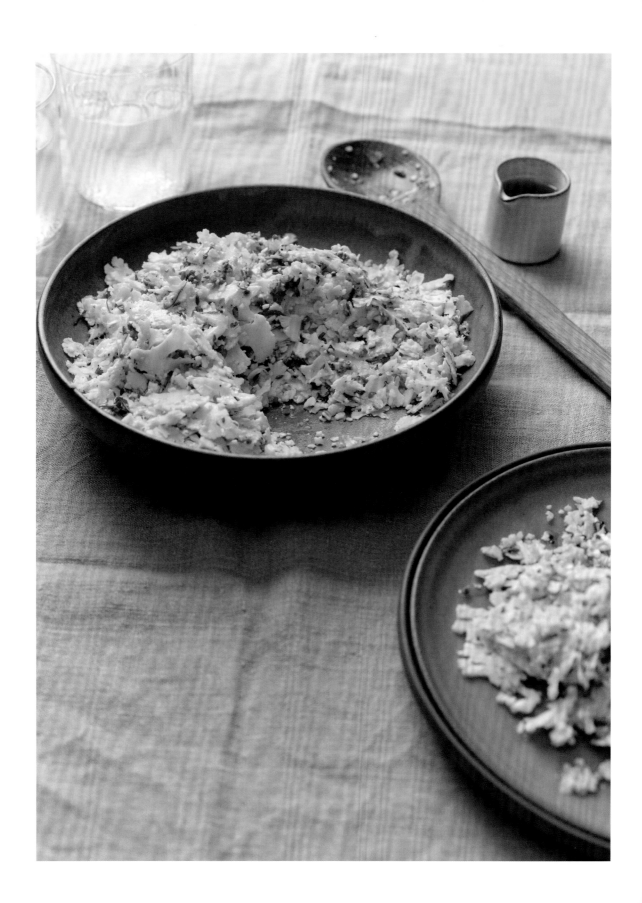

Raw cauliflower salad

Amanda loves raw cauliflower and could eat this every day. If you're not feeling too confident using a mandoline or sharp knife, just use a box grater on the coarsest setting for the cauliflower, and you will still get fantastic results. This is a great accompaniment to my Flattened lamb kebabs (page 130).

Nutrition notes

Cauliflower is certainly a heart-healthy vegetable, thanks to a specific antioxidant compound that is found in plants called sulforaphane. Sulforaphane is higher in raw cruciferous vegetables and is produced when cruciferous vegetables are damaged, so shaving raw cauliflower is an excellent technique to ensure high amounts of this chemical are ingested. Emerging research suggests that because of its antioxidant effects, sulforaphane may benefit heart health by reducing inflammation. Inflammation contributes to raising blood pressure and narrowing arteries – both risk factors for heart disease.

Equipment | A very sharp knife, or invest in a Japanese mandoline

1 Shave the florets of cauliflower wafer thin using the mandoline/knife, then place them into a bowl of iced water and leave for 30 minutes (this will help to crisp up the cauliflower). Drain in a colander and place in a large bowl with the chopped coriander and mint.

2 Whisk all the vinaigrette ingredients in a bowl, then pour over the cauliflower and toss just before serving.

Serves 2

1 small cauliflower, broken into florets
15g (½oz) coriander leaves, chopped
15g (½oz) mint leaves, chopped

For the vinaigrette
100ml (3½fl oz) extra virgin olive oil
20ml (½fl oz) sherry vinegar
1 small shallot, finely sliced
1 small red chilli, finely sliced
1 teaspoon ground toasted cumin seeds
1 teaspoon ground toasted coriander seeds
Juice of 1 lime
Flaked sea salt, to taste

My Asian slaw

This slaw goes with my Salmon XO (page 104) and Cod with miso (page 109) really well. I love all those punchy flavours of the sour and salt from the rice wine vinegar and the nam pla. Make sure you don't dress this dish too early as the dressing will break down the salad and you want it to have plenty of bite.

Nutrition notes

This coleslaw provides a great opportunity to eat a diverse range of vegetables in their raw form. Raw vegetables have a higher nutrient and fibre content compared to cooked, which offers a good healthy option here. Cabbage is often overlooked in favour of other vegetables, but it has an impressive nutrient content, as it is especially high in vitamin C, a potent antioxidant. Antioxidants protect the body from damage caused by free radicals, which are molecules that have an odd number of electrons, making them unstable. When their levels become too high, they can damage the cells in our body. Cabbage is also high in fibre and rich in vitamin B6 and folate, which are important for energy metabolism and support the nervous system.

Equipment | A very sharp knife, or invest in a Japanese mandoline

1. Make the dressing first by whisking everything together and seasoning with salt and pepper, if needed.

2. Place all your salad ingredients in a bowl and mix. Pour over the dressing and mix again - you can use as much or as little as you like. Leave to marinate for up to 30 minutes before serving.

Serves 2

100g (3½oz) Savoy cabbage, sliced wafer thin
100g (3½oz) red cabbage, sliced wafer thin
1 medium carrot, shaved wafer thin
3 spring onions, thinly sliced
½ red pepper, deseeded and thinly sliced
10g (¼oz) fresh coriander, chopped
1 tablespoon toasted sesame seeds
1 bird's eye chilli, finely chopped

For the dressing

50ml (2fl oz) olive oil
15ml (½fl oz) sesame oil
30ml (1fl oz) nam pla
30ml (1fl oz) rice wine vinegar
30ml (1fl oz) soy sauce
10g (¼oz) grated ginger
1 garlic clove, grated
1 teaspoon honey
Juice of ½ lime
Flaked sea salt and freshly ground black pepper, to taste

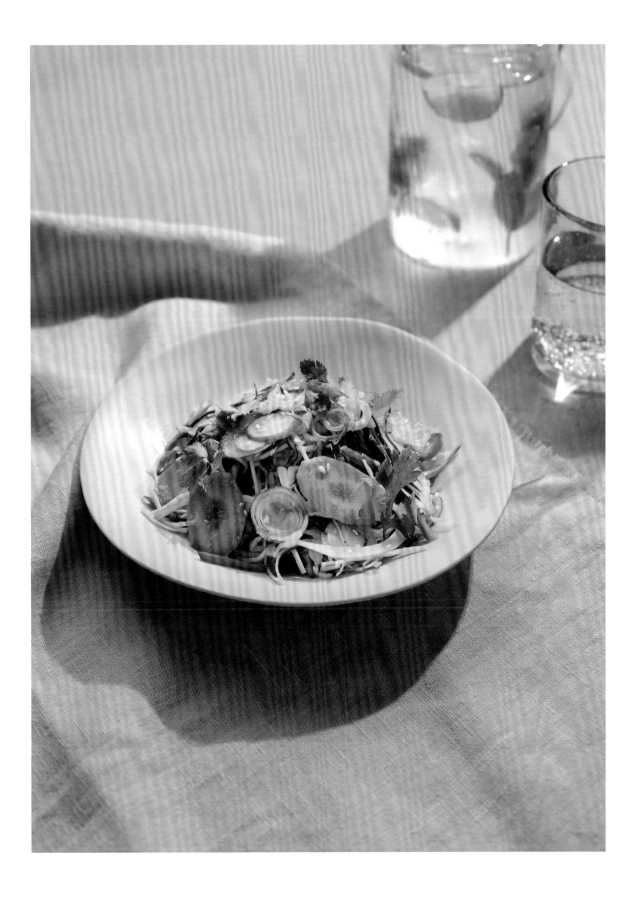

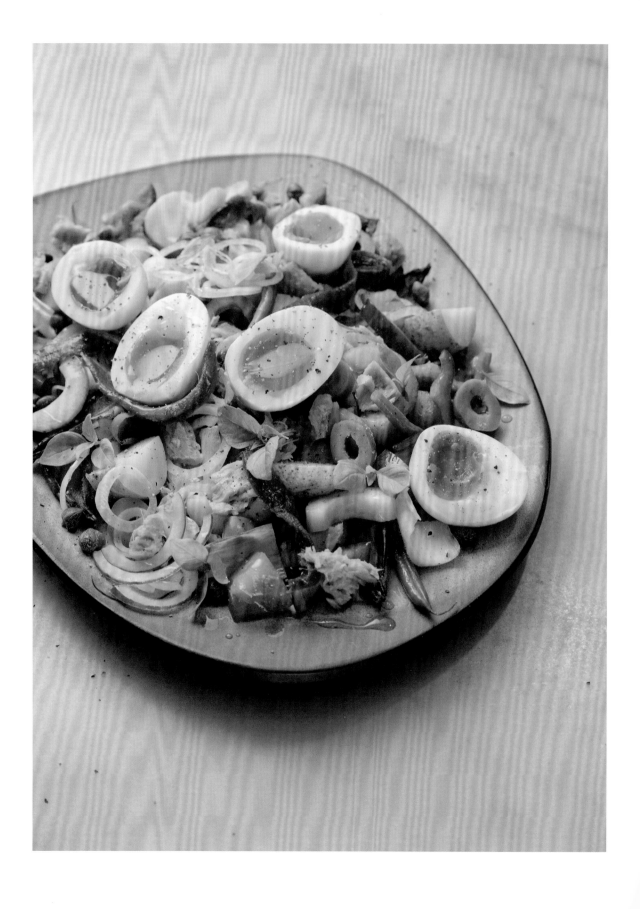

My tuna niçoise

You will notice a lot of my recipes are devised to save you time and energy when plating up, and that's because I cook like this at home all the time, so it becomes a joy to prepare the meal. Also the pressure is off when plating is so simple. I hope this gives you bags of confidence; I like breaking down the preconception of food that sometimes looks too pretty. This food is meant to be eaten....

Nutrition notes

Tuna is an excellent source of protein and B vitamins; eating the tinned version is a convenient way of getting the nutritious goodness of this fish. It also contains an amino acid called taurine. The main biological actions of taurine in the body are to conjugate bile acids and regulate blood pressure, both important regulators for health and risk factors for cardiovascular disease. Therefore, it seems plausible that these mechanisms would suggest that increased taurine intake may be important for improving cardiovascular health. However, data from human intervention studies is limited. Like all the foods in this book, it may be that rather than focusing on one compound from a single food, we should rather view our ingredients as a whole because each have their own unique and diverse nutrient makeup.

Serves 2

2 plum tomatoes, cut into wedges

1 long red pepper, cut into strips

½ medium cucumber, peeled, seeds removed and cut into 2cm (¾in) chunks

1 small red onion, thinly sliced

1 red chicory, cut in half and then into 3cm (1¼in) slices

1 white chicory, cut in half and then into 3cm (1¼in) slices

12 olives, pitted and cut in half

75g French beans, cooked and chilled

1 x 185g (6oz) tin tuna (I use Ortiz), drained and flaked

100g (3½oz) new potatoes, boiled in salted water, chilled and cut in half

15g (½oz) basil leaves, torn (save half to finish)

1 tablespoon capers

1 tablespoon soy sauce

Extra virgin olive oil, for drizzling

4 large organic eggs, boiled for 6 minutes, chilled, shelled and cut in half

Flaked sea salt and freshly ground black pepper, to taste

1   Mix all the ingredients except the oil, boiled eggs and seasoning together in a bowl. Drizzle with the olive oil, and season with salt and pepper.

2   Plate up and top with the egg halves. Drizzle over a little more olive oil and scatter over the reserved basil.

Roast chicken salad, beluga lentils, pickled ginger and sriracha

I use beluga lentils in a pouch, as they are cooked already so it saves loads of prep time (they get their name from their resemblance to beluga caviar). Resting the chicken thighs after cooking allows the meat to become tender and the juices to flow as the meat relaxes. A chef's tip is adding the roasting juices that would usually be discarded, which gives a massive boost of flavour.

Nutrition notes

Lentils are really great source of both soluble and insoluble fibre. A high-fibre diet has been shown to reduce cholesterol and blood pressure, improve digestion, help to lower blood sugar levels and contribute to maintaining a healthy weight. This recipe also includes the Korean favourite, kimchi. There are hundreds of different variants of kimchi, but essentially it is fermented cabbage with many other vegetables and spices. Kimchi is classed as symbiotic food, because the fermentation process results in the production of beneficial probiotic bacteria and the fibre content acts as prebiotic or fertilizer for these beneficial microbes. Regular consumption of kimchi has been shown to increase the quantity of good bacteria in the gut after two weeks and improve indicators of cardiometabolic health.

Serves 2

6 boneless and skinless chicken thighs
30ml (1fl oz) extra virgin olive oil
1 x 250g (9oz) pouch of cooked beluga lentils
Zest and juice of 1 lemon
2 tablespoons kimchi, chopped
1 tablespoon sriracha
10g (¼oz) pickled ginger, thinly sliced
Flaked sea salt and freshly ground black pepper, to taste

1   Preheat the oven to 180°C/400°F/gas mark 6.

2   Place the chicken thighs on a roasting tray and season with a little of the olive oil, salt and pepper. Cook in the oven for 20–30 minutes until golden brown and cooked through.

3   Meanwhile, in a large mixing bowl add the lentils, chopped kimchi, sriracha, pickled ginger, lemon zest and juice. Season with salt and pepper and a drizzle of olive oil, and taste for seasoning.

4   Remove the chicken from the oven and allow to rest and cool for 15 minutes, then cut into thin strips and add to the salad, drizzling over the cooking juices from the roasting tray. Give it a good toss and serve on 2 large plates.

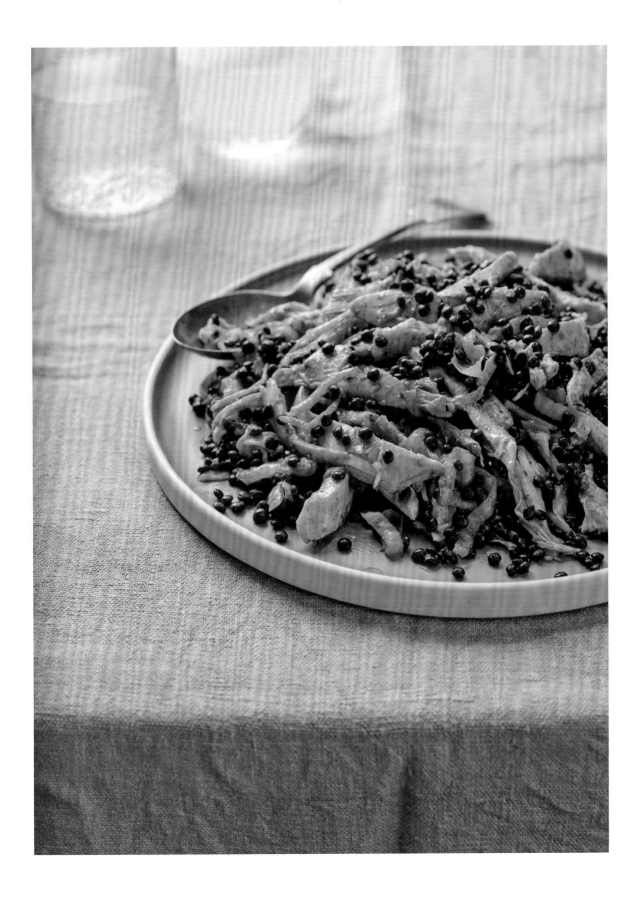

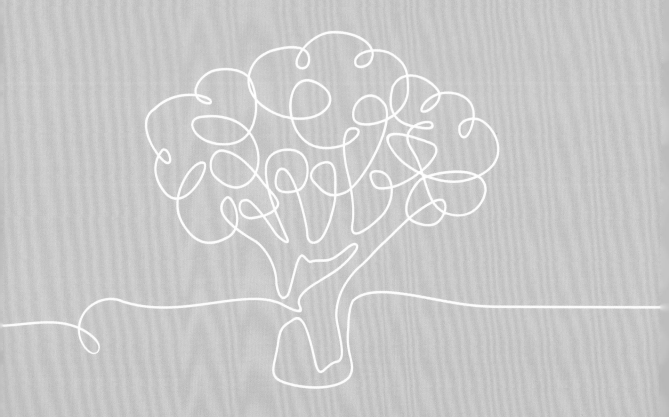

3

vegetables

Momma Bains' chickpea curry

This is one of my growing-up dishes. When we were all in lockdown, we opened up a new company with my mum called Momma Bains; we got Mum to cook all her curries then we made them, step-by-step, with her writing down all the recipes and formulating them. This is one of my favourites, especially with a samosa sitting on top – what I call a 'Punjabi 99', we sell in Wollaton Park every fortnight from our food truck.

Nutrition notes

Chickpeas are an excellent source of carbohydrate, protein, fibre and B vitamins and they are a nutritious staple of many diets. In addition, they have a low glycaemic index and low glycaemic load, and they also contain amylose, which is a resistant starch that is digested slowly. This helps control blood glucose and insulin levels in response to eating and may support blood sugar control in people with type 2 diabetes. From a heart-disease perspective, chickpeas contain a plant sterol called sitosterol. Sitosterol is structurally similar to cholesterol in the body, so it interferes with the body's absorption of cholesterol and can help to lower blood cholesterol levels.

1 Place a saucepan on a medium heat and add the olive oil. When hot, add the shallots, garlic and cumin seeds and cook until the veg is slightly golden, around 20 minutes.

2 Add the tomatoes and bring to a simmer, then add the ginger, chilli and turmeric. Carry on cooking until the oil splits out and the mixture takes on a purée texture. Add the chickpeas and bring to a simmer. Pour in the water, bring back to a simmer and cook for 30 minutes. Remove from the heat, then add the coriander and season with salt.

Serves 2

30ml (1fl oz) extra virgin olive oil
2 shallots, finely diced
15g (½oz) grated garlic
1 tablespoon toasted cumin seeds
200g (7oz) tinned chopped tomatoes
15g (½oz) grated ginger
1 green chilli, sliced
1 teaspoon ground turmeric
200g (7oz) tinned chickpeas, drained
200ml (7fl oz) water
20g (¾oz) fresh coriander, chopped
Flaked sea salt, to taste

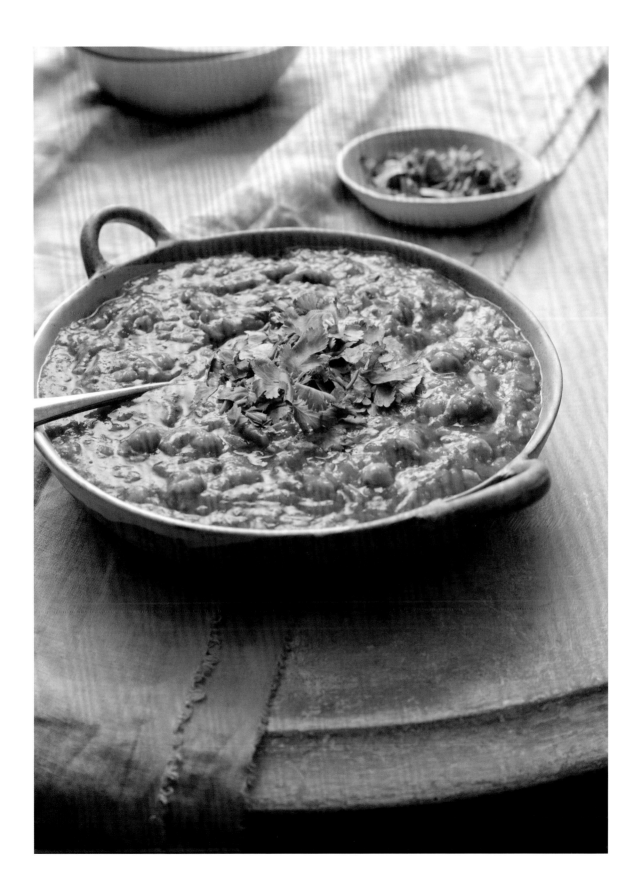

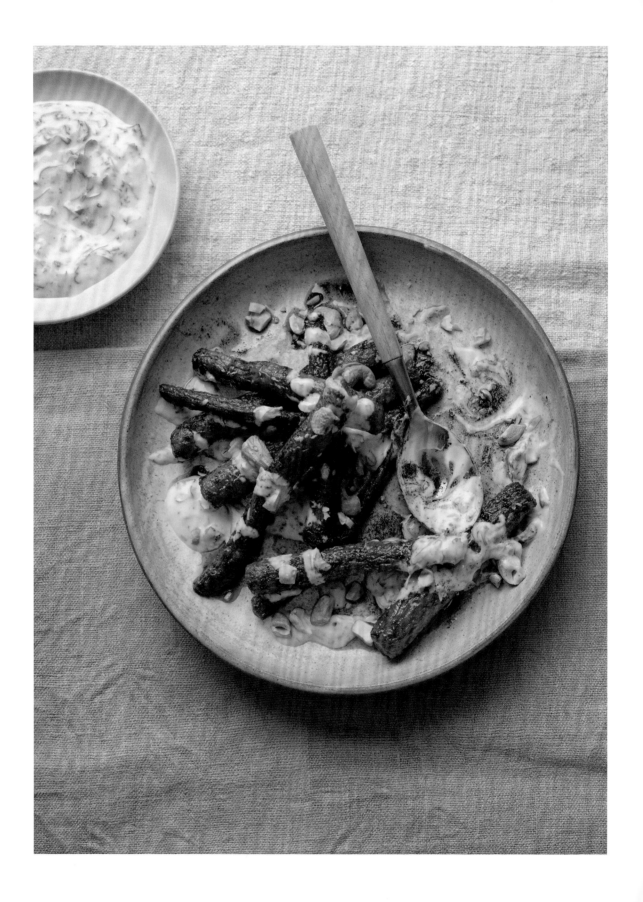

Oven-baked carrots with garam masala, mint, coriander, lime and yoghurt

Carrots are a go-to veg for me, and this recipe is about bringing out their sweetness by adding spices and cooking them slow so the sugars caramelize and the juices amalgamate. You can do this with other roots, too, such as beetroot and parsnips - give them a try and pair them with your favourite meats. I love these with my lamb chops and lamb kebabs.

Nutrition notes

Carrots get both their name and their vibrant orange colour from their high content of the compound called carotenoid. About 80 per cent of the carotenes found in carrots are called beta-carotene and are often referred to as provitamin A, which our gut converts into vitamin A. Most of these carotenoids are found in the flesh and outer root of the carrot. Importantly, studies have shown that when we cook carrots with extra virgin olive oil we can increase the amount of beta-carotene that our body can absorb. In addition to their synonymous association with eye health, carotenoids may also be important for cardiovascular health. Another carotenoid compound known as lycopene can help lower bad (LDL) cholesterol. Subsequently, systematic reviews of the literature suggest that high dietary intakes of lycopene alongside a healthy balanced diet and exercise may support a reduction in risk of cardiovascular disease.

Equipment | A sealable freezer bag

1 Make a paste in a small bowl by combining the garam masala, cumin seeds, olive oil and salt. Transfer to a sealable freezer bag, add the whole carrots and massage the paste all over to evenly coat. Leave for 3 hours to marinate.

2 Mix together all the ingredients for the dressing and leave in the fridge until needed.

3 Preheat the oven to 180°C/400°F/gas mark 6.

4 Place the carrots in a roasting tray and cook in the oven until tender and golden brown, for around 30-45 minutes. Remove from the oven and place the carrots on a serving plate. Spoon over the dressing and top with the toasted cashews.

Serves 2

1 teaspoon garam masala
1 teaspoon toasted cumin seeds
1 tablespoon extra virgin olive oil
Pinch of flaked sea salt
250g (9oz) medium carrots, trimmed
10g (¼oz) toasted and chopped cashew nuts, to serve

For the dressing
150g (5oz) natural yoghurt
5g (⅛oz) mint leaves, finely chopped
5g (⅛oz) coriander leaves, finely chopped
Zest and juice of 1 lime

John's roast aubergine with harissa, chilli and pomegranate molasses

John is my head chef and started with me 22 years ago as a young boy, he has been by my side since and I have seen him grow into a leader, a father and, most of all, a friend. He loves cooking at home as much as I do and we both love this dish: the caramelized aubergines are delicious, the aroma of the natural sugars of the pomegranate molasses cooking on the barbecue is intoxicating, and the seeds are a great addition for the cooling burst of sour pomegranate and their lovely texture.

Nutrition notes

The brilliant deep-purple skin of aubergine is a sign that it is packed full of protective anthocyanin compounds with antioxidant properties. The purple compound nasunin has been shown to help with brain function; and alongside aubergine's high fibre content, this means this vegetable is great at helping to manage bad LDL cholesterol. Nasunin, alongside another aubergine skin compound, chlorogenic acid, can dilate blood vessels, which in turn may help to control blood pressure.

Equipment | Barbecue

1   Place the aubergine quarters on a tray, cut side up, and liberally drizzle over the olive oil and pomegranate molasses. Sprinkle with the harissa powder and lemon zest and leave to marinate for 1 hour.

2   Heat the barbecue. Cook the aubergine pieces on a hot barbecue for around 3 minutes on each side – you want them to be slightly charred. Remove from the barbecue and place back on the tray you used for marinating. Season with the lemon juice, salt and pepper.

3   Top with the chillies, followed by the feta cheese, mint and pomegranate seeds.

Serves 2

1 aubergine, cut into quarters
Extra virgin olive oil, for drizzling
1 tablespoon pomegranate molasses, for drizzling
2 teaspoons dried harissa powder
Zest and juice of 1 lemon
2 long red chillies, finely sliced

50g (2oz) feta cheese, crumbled
Handful of mint leaves, chopped
50g (2oz) pomegranate seeds
Flaked sea salt and freshly ground white pepper, to taste

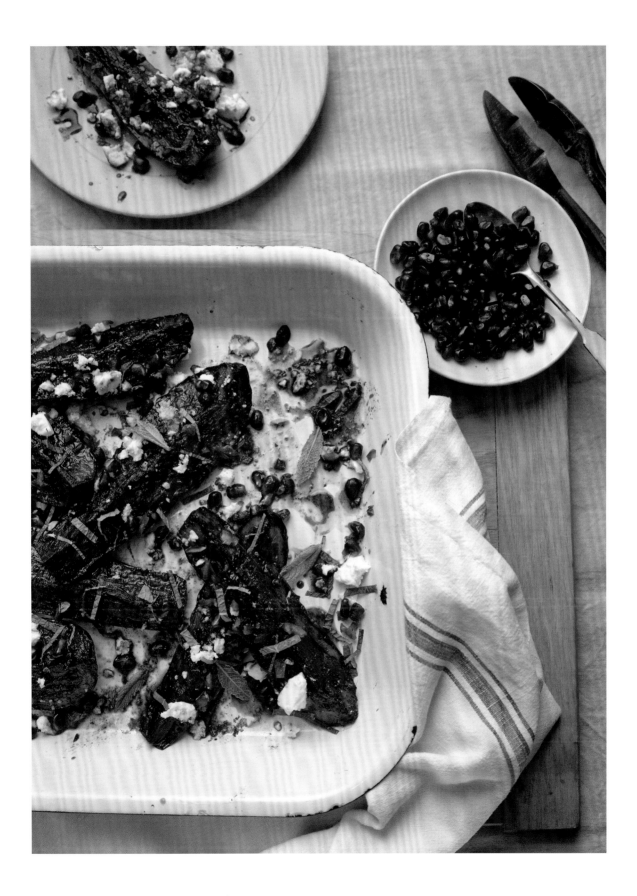

Momma Bains' aubergine and potato sabji

A classic sabji – an Indian term that simply means 'vegetable dish' – in my mum's style. I grew up eating mainly vegetarian curries, and this is one of my faves. The secret of this dish is to pre-cook the potatoes and aubergine dice in an air fryer until tender and golden. I would definitely invest in one for this and so many other dishes, as you need the aubergine to take on a beautiful and toasted hue to release its sugars and become a dark golden colour.

Nutrition notes

Aubergines, famous for their deep-purple skin encasing a light-coloured spongy flesh, are high in fibre, which makes them a valuable addition to a diverse healthy diet, as high-fibre foods can help to manage blood glucose levels. Interestingly, although only evident in test-tube studies currently, extracts of aubergine (phenolic antioxidants) may help control glucose absorption, which is important in the management of diabetes.

Equipment | Air fryer

1 To precook the vegetables, place the aubergine and potatoes in a large bowl, add the extra virgin olive oil, and mix, making sure each vegetable piece is coated. Preheat your air fryer to 190°C/375°F. Place the potatoes in the air fryer and cook for 2–3 minutes, then add the aubergines and cook for a further 10–12 minutes. Remove and set aside.

2 Heat the oil in a pan over a medium heat , then add cumin seeds and toast gently for 1 minute. Add the shallots and cook until translucent, around 10 minutes.

3 Add the garlic, ginger and chilli and cook for a further 10 minutes.

4 Add the tomatoes and bring to a simmer, then carry on cooking for around 30 minutes. At this point the mixture should have thickened a little. Now fold in the precooked aubergine and potatoes.

5 Remove from the heat and add the fenugreek, then season and sprinkle with the coriander to finish.

Serves 2

300g (10oz) aubergine, cut into 4cm (1½in) dice
200g (7oz) potatoes, cut into 3cm (1¼in) dice
75ml (3fl oz) extra virgin olive oil, plus 1 tablespoon for air frying
1 tablespoon cumin seeds
2 shallots, finely diced
15g (½oz) grated garlic
15g (½oz) grated ginger
1 green chilli, finely diced
150g (5oz) tinned chopped tomatoes
5g (⅛oz) chopped fenugreek
10g (¼oz) fresh coriander, chopped, to serve
Flaked sea salt, to taste

Brussels sprout sabji

This is one of Amanda's and my favourite sabjis that my mum makes in winter. The lovely nutty flavour that the sprouts bring really lend themselves to the curry method. I also like this cold in sandwiches with leftover roast turkey.

Nutrition notes

Brussels sprouts are part of the brassica family, along with broccoli and kale, and these small, green, edible buds provide a depth of nutrients that can support a heart-healthy diet. They are incredibly rich in antioxidants, which are protective compounds that reduce oxidative stress in your cells, and as a result may help lower your risk of chronic disease. One research study showed that eating 300g (10oz) of Brussels sprouts a day for three weeks (yes, that's a lot!) reduced oxidative damage. That is not likely to be sustainable, but including Brussels in a diverse diet will also increase our intake of the plant compound called kaempferol, which studies suggest could support hearth health.

1   Heat 15ml (½fl oz) of the oil in a large saucepan until hot, then add the Brussels sprouts and cook for 4–5 minutes until caramelized. Remove from the pan and transfer to kitchen paper to drain.

2   Place the pan on a medium-high heat and add the remaining 100ml (3¼fl oz) of oil. Add the onions, ginger, garlic and chilli and cook until the moisture from the onions has evaporated. Lower the heat to medium and gently cook for around 1 hour until the mix is golden brown.

3   Add the turmeric, tomatoes and water and bring to a simmer, then add the Brussels sprouts and cook for 20 minutes.

4   Add the fenugreek and season with salt, then remove from the heat and stir in the coriander to serve.

Serves 2

115ml (3¾fl oz) extra virgin olive oil
280g (9½oz) Brussels sprouts, cut into quarters
150g (5oz) Spanish onions, finely sliced
25g (1oz) grated ginger
25g (1oz) grated garlic
20g (¾oz) green chilli, finely sliced
10g (¼oz) ground turmeric
100g (3½oz) tinned chopped tomatoes
100ml (3½fl oz) water
10g (¼oz) chopped fenugreek
Flaked sea salt, to taste
25g (1oz) fresh coriander, chopped, to serve

Baked courgette, fennel seeds, olive oil and anchovies

Dishes like this make a brilliant alternative to the veg served for a Sunday roast, and courgettes can easily be interchanged with aubergine. The dressing is full of punchy flavours and when drizzled over the cooked courgettes, their heat will release the perfumes and flavours of the anchovies and lemon.

Nutrition notes

Courgettes are part of the cucurbit family of plants, which also includes cucumbers and squash, amongst many others. Although courgettes have a high water content, they still have plenty of nutritious content, with significant amounts of potassium, folate and vitamins A and C. Furthermore, due to their polysaccharide content they may support lowering of LDL cholesterol and managing blood sugar levels.

Serves 2

250g (9oz) courgette, sliced at an angle 3cm (1in) thick
Extra virgin olive oil, for brushing
10g (¼oz) sprigs of thyme
Flaked sea salt and freshly ground black pepper, to taste

For the dressing
1 teaspoon toasted fennel seeds
1 tablespoon extra virgin olive oil
4 anchovies (I use Ortiz), chopped
Juice of 1 lemon
1 tablespoon toasted pine nuts
5g (⅛oz) basil leaves, torn
1 teaspoon pomegranate molasses

1   Preheat the oven to 200°C/425°F/gas mark 7.

2   Lay out the courgette slices on a roasting tray. Brush olive oil on both sides of the courgette, season with salt and pepper and add the thyme sprigs. Place in the oven and cook until golden brown, 10-15 minutes each side.

3   Mix all the ingredients together for the dressing in a bowl and set aside.

4   When the courgettes are cooked, remove from the oven and place on a serving plate. Drizzle the dressing all over and serve.

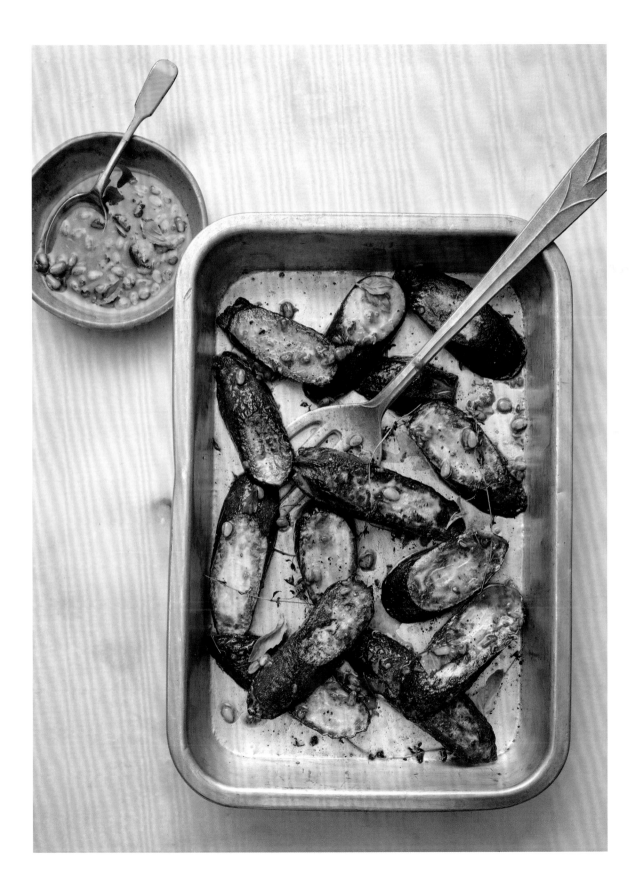

Lentil dhal

Being born into a Punjabi household meant there was often an aroma of curry, garlic and steamed spinach in the house. I hated it at the time, but now, as a grown man, I love it - they are the smells and flavours of my youth, the pulses and dhals that Mum cooked when I was growing up. I never knew they were so healthy, nor realized that 60 per cent of my childhood was spent eating plant-based vegetarian food, which also always tasted better the next day. Asians tend to cook with a lot of ghee and have a predisposition to heart disease, so by eliminating the traditional ghee and using olive oil here instead, this really does bring this recipe into line with a health-conscious diet.

Nutrition notes

Lentils are a great choice for a heart-healthy diet, and are included in number of recipes within the book, so for detail on the nutritional power of the little lentil see the recipes on pages 58 and 152.

1   Tip the lentils into a sieve and rinse under cold running water. Drain and set aside.

2   Heat the olive oil in a pan on a medium heat until hot, then add the onions and cook for 2-3 minutes until softened. Add the ginger, garlic and chilli and cook over a high heat for 5-6 minutes, making sure all the moisture has evaporated. Lower the heat to the lowest setting and cook for another 20 minutes, you are trying to get as much moisture out and allowing the natural sugars to sweeten the base mix.

3   Add the lentils and stir in the turmeric, give it a good mix, then add the water. Bring to a simmer and cook for about 20 minutes or until the lentils are cooked and all the water has evaporated. Season with a little salt, then add the garam masala. Remove from the heat and stir in the coriander.

Serves 2

125g (4½oz) dried red
   lentils
100g (3½oz) extra virgin
   olive oil
100g (3½oz) Spanish
   onions, finely sliced
15g (½oz) ginger, grated
20g (¾oz) garlic, grated
10g (¼oz) green chilli,
   finely sliced
1 teaspoon ground
   turmeric
875ml (1½ pints) water
1 teaspoon garam masala
Flaked sea salt, to taste
20g (¾oz) fresh coriander,
   chopped, to serve

Roasted root vegetables, rosemary, garlic and ras el hanout

Roasting root vegetables is one of my favourite ways to serve them; I love the way they caramelize and how the natural sugars mix with the spices to create an incredible flavour. When combined with the famous duo of rosemary and garlic, they bring a lovely earthiness to the whole dish. This would go perfectly with my Lamb chops with harissa on page 127.

This would go perfectly with my Lamb chops with harissa on page 127.

⊕ **Nutrition notes**

Roasting the vegetables in this recipe provides a fantastic opportunity to combine a range of fresh tasty roots with delicious herbs and spices. Research has shown that people who eat seven or more portions of fruit and vegetables a day have the lowest risk of mortality from any cause, with vegetables having significantly higher health benefits than fruit. Furthermore, increasing vegetable intake not only improves physical health but has been shown to improve psychological wellbeing by increasing feelings of happiness too. So eat the rainbow and feel better both inside and out.

Serves 2

1 large parsnip
1 large carrot
1 small celeriac
1 small turnip
1 red potato
1 bulb of garlic, split in half widthways, skin on
2 red onions, each cut into three
Large pinch of flaked sea salt
10g (¼oz) ras el hanout
1 small sprig of rosemary, leaves picked
1 teaspoon freshly ground black pepper
100ml (3½fl oz) olive oil

1   Preheat the oven to 180°C/400°F/gas mark 6 with a large non-stick, deep-sided oven tray inside.

2   Wash all the root vegetables and pat dry with kitchen paper, but do not peel. Cut each vegetable into as equal sizes as you can to leave them all quite chunky and robust.

3   In a large bowl combine all the vegetables with the sea salt, ras el hanout, rosemary and pepper. Add the olive oil to the bowl and toss the vegetables so they are all well coated in the spice and seasonings.

4   Transfer to the hot tray in the oven and roast for about 45 minutes, turning them every 10 minutes. Once cooked, leave to slightly cool before serving.

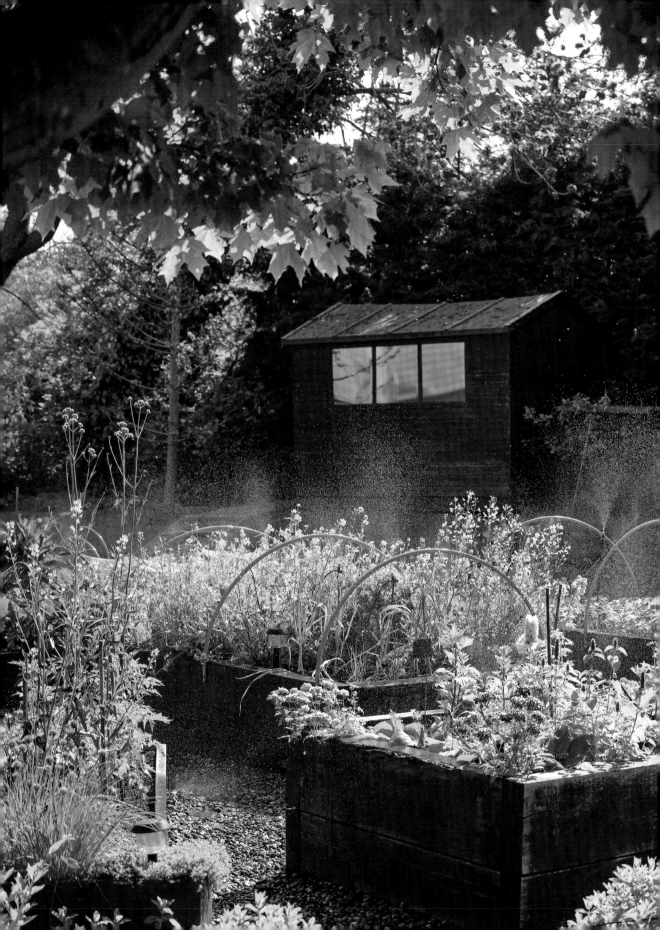

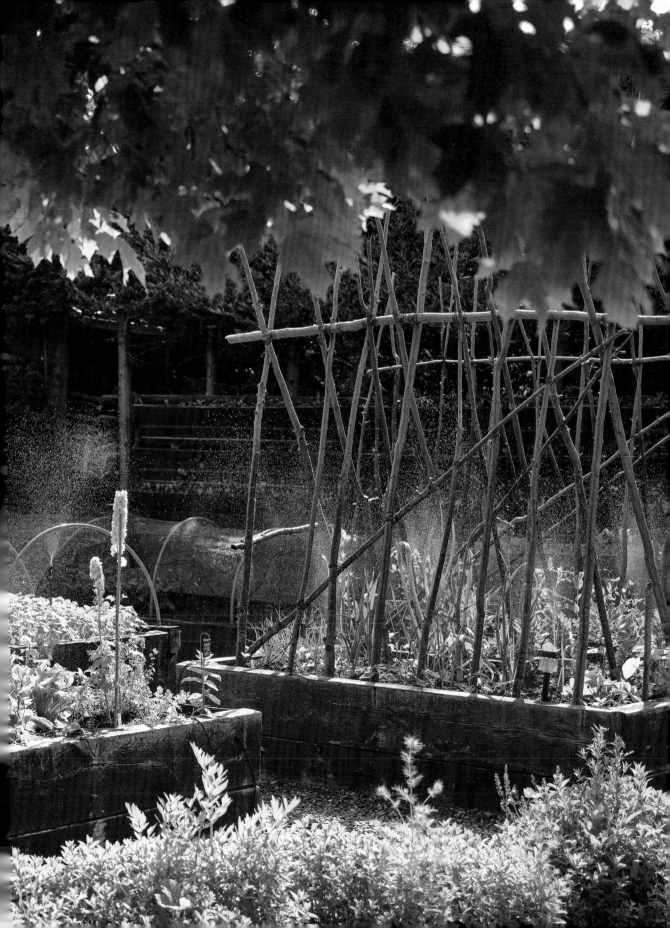

Broccoli with spring onions, chilli, soy and sesame seeds

I eat broccoli most days and try to find lots of ways to keep it exciting, as boredom is the number one reason for why we go back to our old ways and then, before you know it, we start eating rubbish. This Asian-inspired recipe is very high in flavours so it will always excite. I do a lot of recipes this way, where the dressing is made earlier in a large bowl and when the vegetables are cooked they are simply drained and thrown straight into the bowl. Doing it this way means the vegetables heat up the dressing and all its volatile compounds come alive.

Nutrition notes

Broccoli is one of the most popular vegetables from the brassica family, and it is a very nutritious option, with a growing body of evidence that it can have a number of health benefits. Eating steamed broccoli on a regular basis has been suggested to help reduce the risk of cardiovascular disease, due to its ability to lower LDL cholesterol. Furthermore, recent evidence also suggests that broccoli extract can reduce inflammation in human fat cells, which may (further research warranted!) reduce the risk of obesity and type 2 diabetes. Broccoli gets its mild bitter taste from a phytochemical called sulforaphane. In laboratory studies, sulforaphane has been shown to reduce the risk of certain cancers by enhancing the detoxication of carcinogens.

1   Combine all the ingredients for the dressing in a large bowl and set aside.

2   Cook the broccoli in a pan of boiling water for 3–4 minutes or until tender when pierced with the tip of a sharp knife. When cooked, drain and transfer to the bowl with the dressing. Mix well and tip into a serving bowl. Scatter over the spring onions and serve.

Serves 2

250g (9oz) long-stem broccoli
2 spring onions, finely sliced, to serve

For the dressing
1 teaspoon soy sauce
½ teaspoon toasted black sesame seeds
½ teaspoon toasted white sesame seeds
1 teaspoon sesame oil
½ teaspoon dried chilli flakes

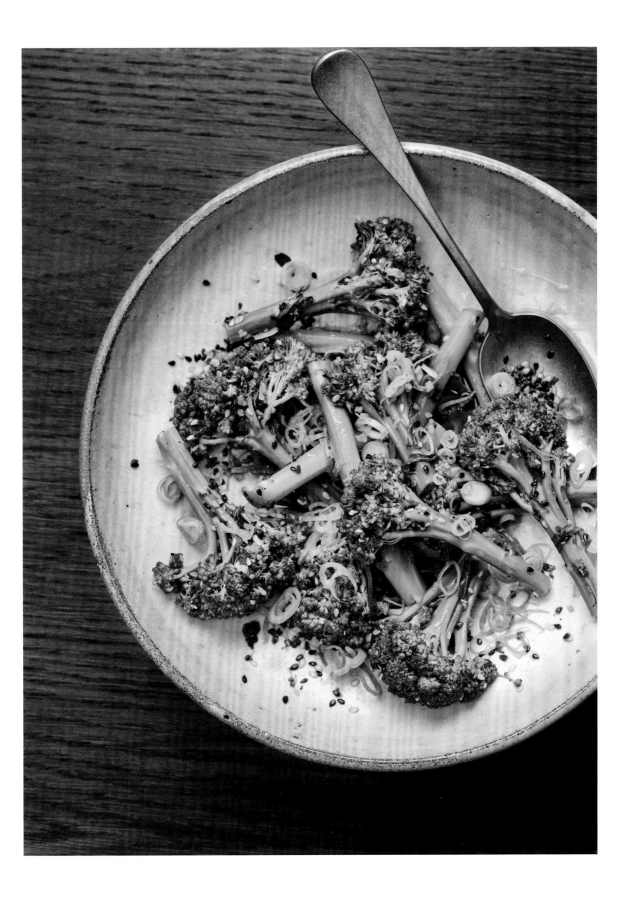

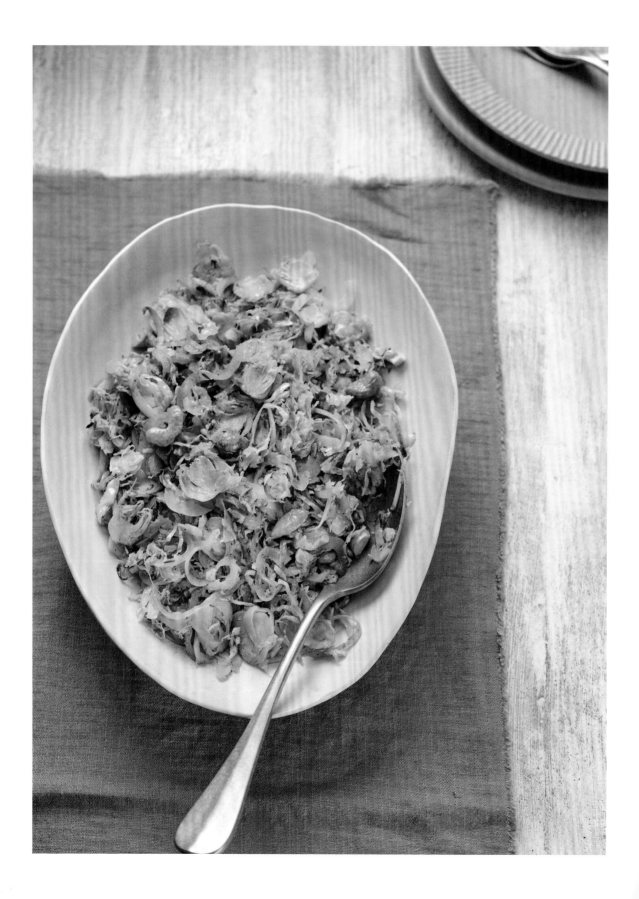

Stir-fried Brussels sprouts with cumin and cashews

This stir-fry is a brilliant, quick and simple dish. The key to success to this and all my recipes is preparing all the ingredients in advance, because this dish is so quick, you don't want to stop the flow of each stage. Also be careful on the seasoning of the salt, as soy sauce is quite intense, so always season at the end of cooking. The cashew and cumin give this dish great texture and aroma. You could always play around and add peanuts and even beansprouts to give it a more textural difference, and always make sure there is a little bite left in the sprouts, too, for a little crunch.

Nutrition notes

Brussels sprouts might not be everyone's favourite vegetable but these little green buds are full of beneficial nutrients and can support the production of glutathione, an antioxidant that also plays an important role in strengthening our gut lining.

Equipment | Wok

1   Heat a large wok on a medium-high heat. Add both oils and allow to heat up. Toss in the sprouts and cook for at least 3 minutes, stirring continuously. Add the onions and cook for 1 minute. Add the chillies, garlic and ginger and cook for 30 seconds, then remove from the heat.

2   Add the soy sauce, cashew nuts and cumin seeds and season with a little salt and pepper. Serve.

Serves 2

20ml (¾fl oz) sesame oil
10ml (¼fl oz) extra virgin olive oil
300g (10oz) Brussels sprouts, thinly sliced
1 medium white onion, thinly sliced
2 red chillies, thinly sliced
10g (¼oz) grated garlic
10g (¼oz) grated ginger

2 tablespoons soy sauce
10g (¼oz) toasted cashew nuts, coarsely chopped
1 teaspoon toasted cumin seeds
Flaked sea salt and freshly ground black pepper, to taste

Spiced sweet potato fries

So quick and so simple, this recipe can also be made with normal potatoes and other roots. I use an air fryer at home; it is such an easy and healthier way to fry and it is one of my best investments. I would definitely recommend purchasing one. If you haven't got an air fryer, don't worry; just cook in a preheated oven set at 180°C/400°F/gas mark 6 for about 20 minutes or until they reach the desired crispiness for you.

Nutrition notes

The sweet potato, with its thin brown skin and often bright-orange flesh, is not actually related to our traditional white potato. It has a superior nutrition content and so is an excellent addition to a diverse diet. Sweet potatoes are particularly high in fibre, which is important for supporting our digestive health. And although no definitive conclusion can be made yet, there is some evidence to suggest that eating sweet potato may help manage blood sugar levels in type 2 diabetes.

Equipment | Air fryer

1   Mix together the smoked paprika, chilli powder, cumin seeds, sumac and sea salt. Place the matchsticks into a bowl and drizzle with olive oil, then sprinkle over the spice mix, making sure to coat each piece of sweet potato.

2   Preheat the air fryer to 200°C/400°F. Lay out the matchsticks on a piece of foil and add to the air fryer. Cook for 8-12 minutes.

Serves 2

1 teaspoon smoked paprika
½ teaspoon chilli powder
½ teaspoon cumin seeds
½ teaspoon sumac
½ teaspoon flaked sea salt
2 medium sweet potatoes,
    cut into thick matchsticks
Extra virgin olive oil

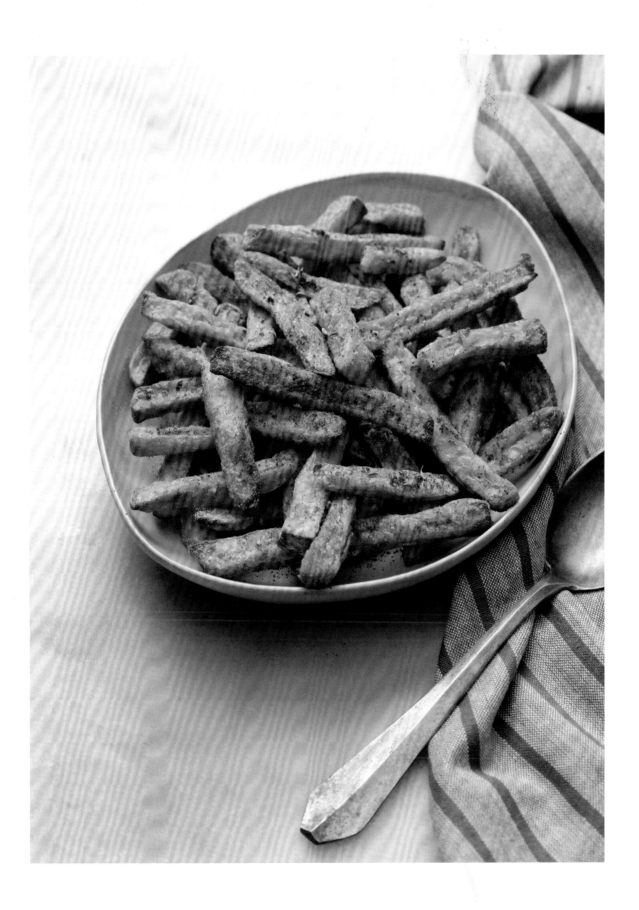

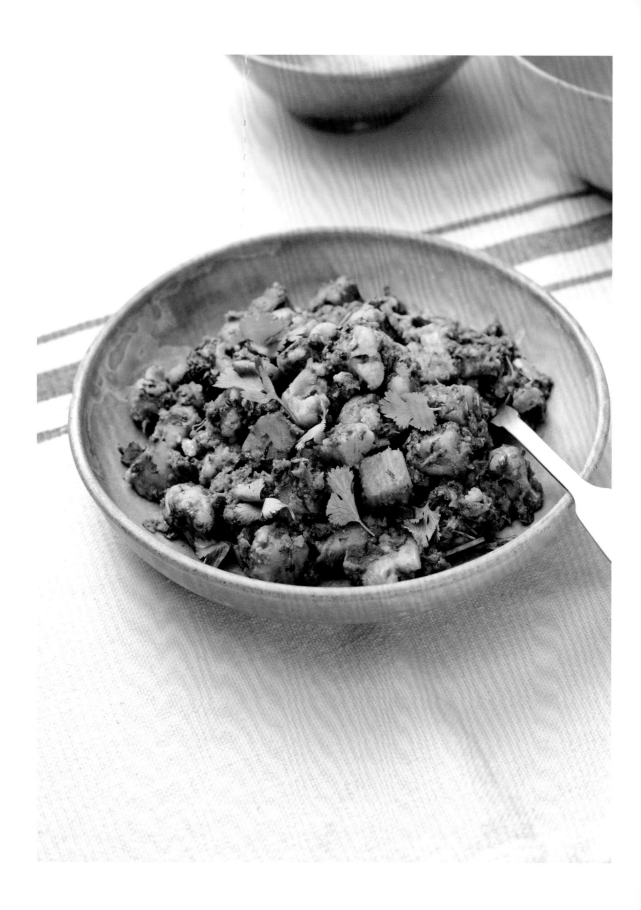

Momma Bains' aloo gobi

Another one of my childhood favourites, my mum's aloo gobi. When I was growing up, Mum wasn't a great cook: she worked full-time and looked after my dad's family and us - around 15 of us - and when we moved and there were just 6 of us, she still wasn't great. But interestingly, when we all left home, she would cook from the heart as all her kids were coming back home for a family catch up and meal and so she introduced a new ingredient into her food: love. Since then, Mum's food has become wholesome, delicious and made with love. So please give this recipe a go.

🫀 Nutrition notes
The fantastic thing about traditional Punjabi cooking is that it's packed full of vegetables, herbs and spices, providing ample opportunity to consume a diverse range of health-supporting compounds. Within this recipe you have the opportunity to eat ginger, garlic, turmeric and tomatoes, which all provide bioactive compounds such as polyphenolic compounds, organosulfur compounds, vitamins, carotenes, curcumin and lycopene. As we have seen in other recipes, these compounds can confer a health benefit when consumed in adequate amounts as part of a diverse and varied diet. For more info on the heart-healthy benefits of cauliflower see the Raw cauliflower salad on page 53.

1   Heat the olive oil in a large saucepan until hot, then add the onions and cook for 2-3 minutes until softened. Turn the heat down to medium and add the ginger, garlic and chilli, and cook for around 30 minutes.

2   Add the water, tomatoes and turmeric and bring to a gentle simmer, then cook for 10 minutes.

3   Add the potatoes and cook until tender, for around 10 minutes. Add the cauliflower and garam masala and cook until tender, for another 10 minutes.

4   Season with a little salt, then remove from the heat and stir in the coriander.

Serves 2

50ml (2fl oz) extra virgin olive oil

100g (3½oz) Spanish onions, finely sliced

15g (½oz) grated ginger

20g (¾oz) grated garlic

10g (¼oz) green chillies, finely sliced

100ml (3½fl oz) water

60g (2oz) fresh chopped tomatoes

¼ teaspoon ground turmeric

200g (7oz) potatoes, peeled and cut into 1½cm (⅝in) dice

200g (7oz) cauliflower florets, cut into bite-size pieces

¼ teaspoon garam masala

20g (¾oz) fresh coriander, chopped, to serve

Flaked sea salt, to taste

Crushed potatoes with feta, olives and capers

Potatoes are most people's go-to vegetables for comfort - think chips, mash and so forth. This recipe lightly crushes the potatoes so they are still intact, but you are basically creating a gnarly surface area that, once roasted in a pan, creates lovely crusty bits that add texture to the dish.

Very much Greek-inspired, all the flavours of this dish merge well and give such diverse elements; the chopped walnuts were a revelation for me when I did this as they work brilliantly, but you can also use pine nuts.

Nutrition notes

Potatoes may be referred to as 'humble', but eating them unprocessed with skin on in this recipe allows them to show off their nutrition credentials. As they are go-to carbohydrates some may have a negative view on the health credentials of potatoes but compared to pasta and rice, gram for gram they can contribute more useful micronutrients to our diet, including vitamin C, folate and potassium.

Serves 2

250g (9oz) new potatoes, skin on
Extra virgin olive oil, for frying

For the dressing
100g (3½oz) barrel-aged feta, cut into 1cm (½in) cubes
16 pitted Kalamata olives, cut into quarters
5g (⅛oz) basil leaves, torn
1 tablespoon capers, drained
20g (¾oz) toasted walnuts, chopped
2 tablespoons extra virgin olive oil
Zest of 1 lemon
Flaked sea salt and freshly ground black pepper, to taste

1   Mix all the ingredients for the dressing, apart from the lemon zest, in a large bowl and set aside.

2   Cook the potatoes in a pan of boiling salted water until tender. Drain, then return to the dry pan and crush gently using the back of a fork.

3   Heat the oil in a frying pan over a medium heat, then add the potatoes and cook on both sides until golden brown and crispy, around 5-6 minutes on each side. Remove from the pan and drain on kitchen paper.

4   Add the potatoes to the dressing, mix well to thoroughly coat, add the lemon zest, then serve.

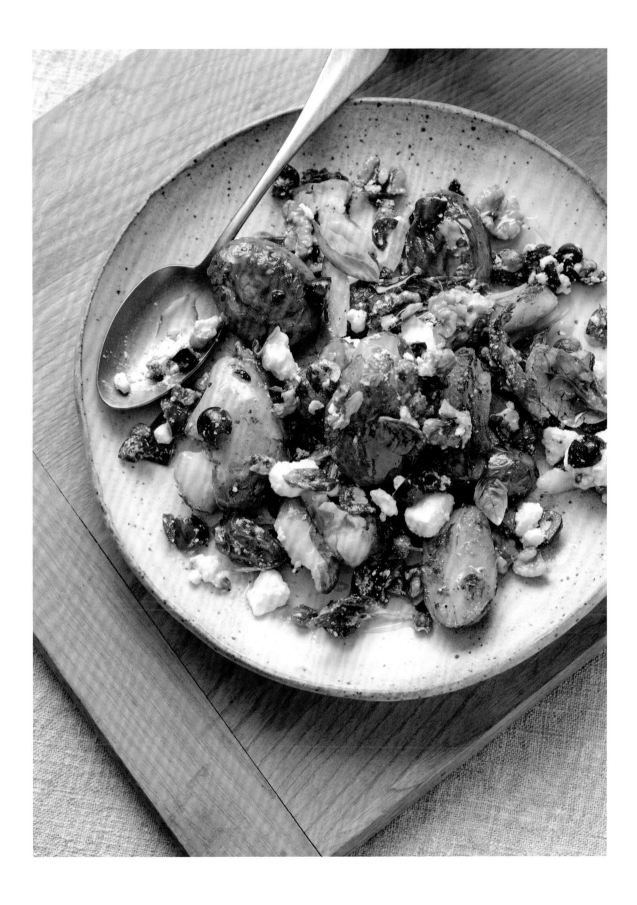

Roasted beetroot with feta, mint and caraway seeds

This recipe is a great way to cook beetroot, it's super simple and delicious. This also works with most root vegetables, so have a go using others and mix up the spices.

🫀 **Nutrition notes**

There is good evidence that beetroot is very effective at increasing nitric oxide availability in the body, and this has emerged as a potential strategy in managing hypertension (raised blood pressure) and supporting endothelial function (endothelium is a thin membrane that lines the inside of the heart and blood vessels). Studies have shown that drinking beetroot juice can preserve endothelial function and lower blood pressure, providing primary evidence for the use of beetroot in a heart-healthy diet.

Serves 2

300g (10oz) beetroot, washed and quartered
75ml (3fl oz) olive oil
1 teaspoon toasted caraway seeds
100g (3½oz) barrel-aged feta cheese
5g (⅛oz) mint leaves
Flaked sea salt and freshly ground black pepper, to taste

1 Preheat the oven to 180°C/400°F/gas mark 6.

2 In a large mixing bowl add the beetroot, olive oil, caraway seeds and some salt and pepper and mix well. Transfer to a roasting tray and cook for about 50 minutes until tender – pierce the beetroot with a sharp knife and it should easily go through.

3 Once cooked, leave the beetroot to cool slightly, then place into a serving bowl. Crumble over the feta and scatter the chopped mint over the whole dish.

Barbecue potatoes with oregano, olive oil and goat's cheese

I love these bad boys in summer when the barbecue is constantly on. The flavour of barbecuing potatoes is something else. The goat's cheese adds a fresh acidity, and it goes all lovely and creamy when combined with the hot potatoes.

Equipment | Barbecue | 20cm (8in) barbecue pan

1   Heat your barbecue.

2   Cook the potatoes in a pan of salted boiling water until tender.

3   Meanwhile, place the goat's cheese, pine nuts, lemon zest and juice, oregano and olive oil in a bowl and gently mix.

4   Drain the potatoes, then return them to the dry pan and gently crush them using the back of a fork. Carefully transfer the potatoes to the barbecue pan and drizzle with a little olive oil. Season with salt and pepper and place the pan on the barbecue grill.

51   Cook the potatoes until they are golden brown and slightly charred. Remove from the barbecue and gently toss them in the bowl with the goat's cheese mixture to coat, then serve while hot.

Serves 2

250g (9oz) new potatoes
100g (3½oz) ripe goat's cheese, cut into 1cm (½in) pieces
100g (3½oz) toasted pine nuts
Zest and juice of 1 lemon
10g (¼oz) sprigs of oregano, leaves picked
1 tablespoon extra virgin olive oil
Flaked sea salt and freshly ground black pepper, to taste

Baked butternut squash, olive oil and Parmesan

This is a great way to eat squash, drizzled with olive oil and sprinkled with its best mate Parmesan and then baked in the oven until tender. The grated lemon accentuates the squash's flavour, too. I would have this with my Peppered pork chop with mustard on page 133.

on page 133.

Nutrition notes

An aim for all of us is to consume as vibrant and diverse a mix of coloured vegetables as possible to ensure we are consuming a range of health-benefiting compounds that are responsible for these colours. Vegetables from the cucurbits family (squashes, marrows, cucumbers, gourds) come in all shapes and colours and therefore provide a great opportunity to do just that. Butternut squash is not only super tasty, but also super nutritious, full of essential vitamins (including vitamins A and C), minerals (including potassium and magnesium), fibre and antioxidants. The carotenoid compounds that give butternut squash its vibrant yellow/orange colour are proposed to help heart health by lowering blood pressure, reducing inflammation and controlling the activity of genes related to heart disease.

1   Preheat the oven to 180°C/400°F/gas mark 6.

2   Place the squash cut side up on a large roasting tray; make sure you leave the skin on as this keeps it all together. Drizzle the olive oil all over both halves and season with salt and pepper. Cook for 40–50 minutes or until the squash has taken on a lovely golden colour and is soft when you place the tip of a knife through it.

3   Remove from the oven and sprinkle the lemon zest over the squash, then grate over the Parmesan until the squash is fully covered. Leave to rest for 5 minutes and then cut into chunks 4–6cm (1½–2½in) across and serve. Don't eat the skin, just scoop out spoonfuls of the tender flesh.

Serves 2

1 medium butternut squash, quartered lengthways, seeds removed
50ml (2fl oz) olive oil
Zest of 1 lemon
50g (2oz) aged Parmesan
Flaked sea salt and freshly ground black pepper, to taste

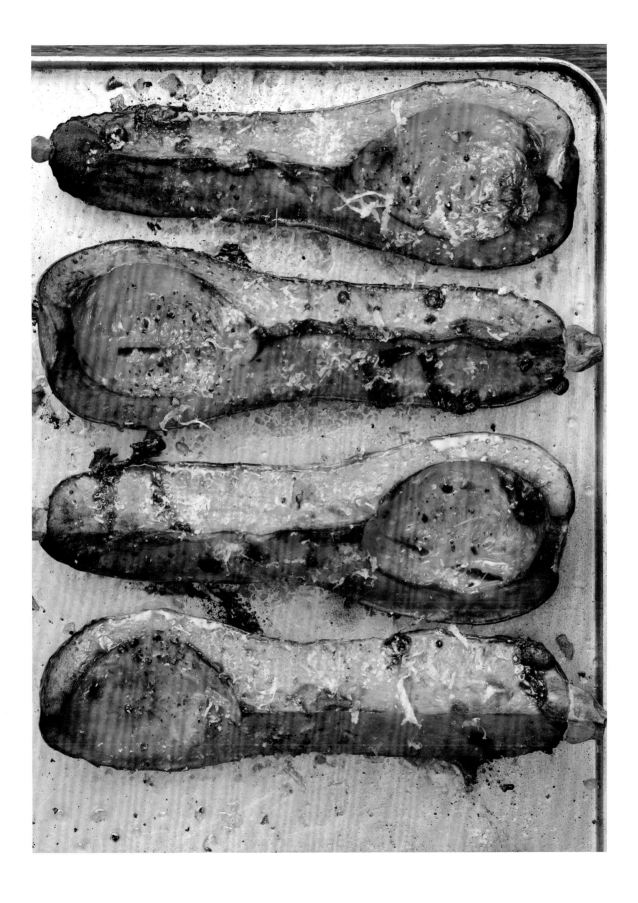

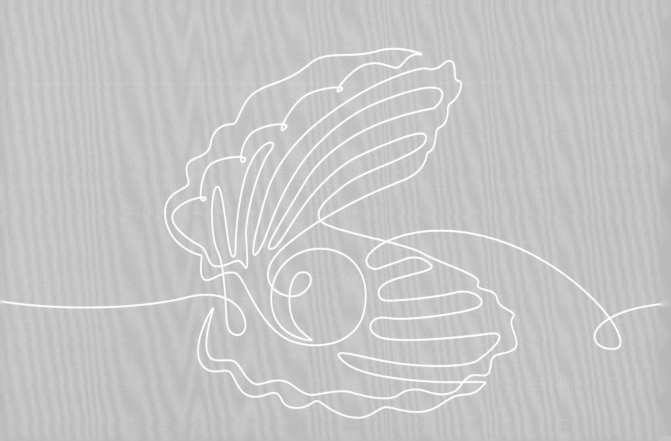

4

fish

Baked salmon with wholemeal penne, lemon and rocket

I think baking salmon is easily one of the most delicate ways to cook it, as it becomes lovely and soft and just breaks into large flakes full of moisture under very little pressure. Buy the best salmon you can find that has certification of not being mass-produced – I use Loch Duart. It is important to work to some timings with this recipe, so that the whole dish comes together at the same time, such as while the salmon is cooking, the pan of water should be on with the pasta cooking too.

🫁 **Nutrition notes**
Salmon is such a great choice of fish to use in cooking to support health. There are a number of recipes in this book using salmon, so please see page 104 for more detail.

Serves 2

500g (1lb 2oz) skinless organic salmon fillets
30ml (1fl oz) olive oil
250g (9oz) wholemeal penne pasta
100g (3½oz) rocket, washed
20g (¾oz) toasted pine nuts
Zest and juice of 1 lemon
50g (2oz) grated Parmesan, plus extra to serve
Nutmeg, for grating
Flaked sea salt and freshly ground black pepper, to taste

1   Preheat the oven to 90°C/400°F/gas mark ¼.

2   Place the salmon on a non-stick tray with a drizzle of the oil and a pinch of salt and cook in the oven for 15–20 minutes. The salmon should still be a little translucent but give when pressed gently. Once the salmon is cooked, gently break it into a bowl into large flakes.

3   Meanwhile, bring a large pan of salted water to a simmer and cook the pasta for 8–10 minutes or as required, leaving it a little al dente.

4   In a large bowl, combine the rocket, pine nuts, lemon zest and juice, salt and pepper and grated Parmesan.

5   The pasta should now be cooked, so drain and while still very hot, add it straight to the bowl and stir gently – the heat will wilt the rocket and liven up the lemon zest. Gently stir in the salmon.

6   Serve in 2 bowls with a drizzle of the olive oil, some more Parmesan and a grating of nutmeg.

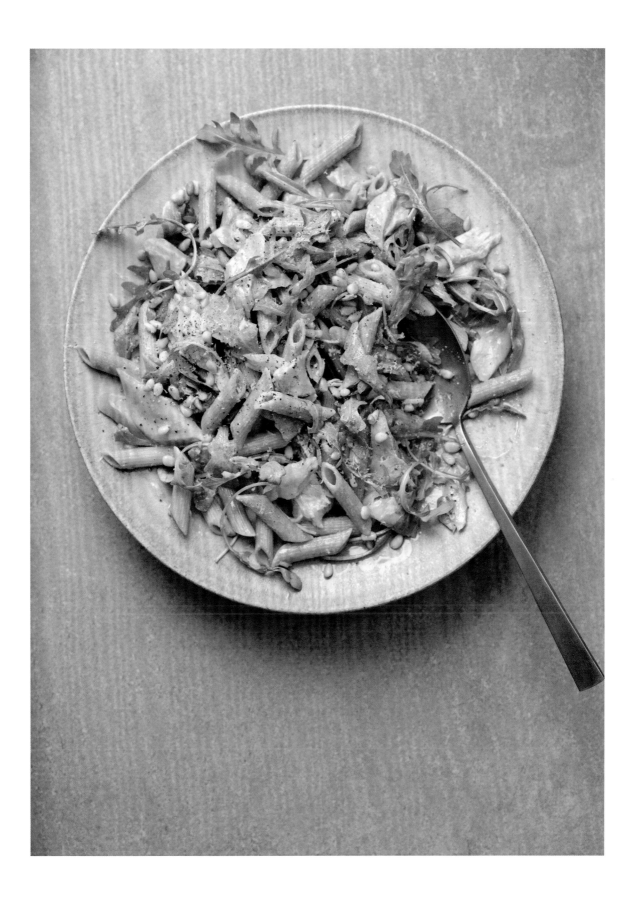

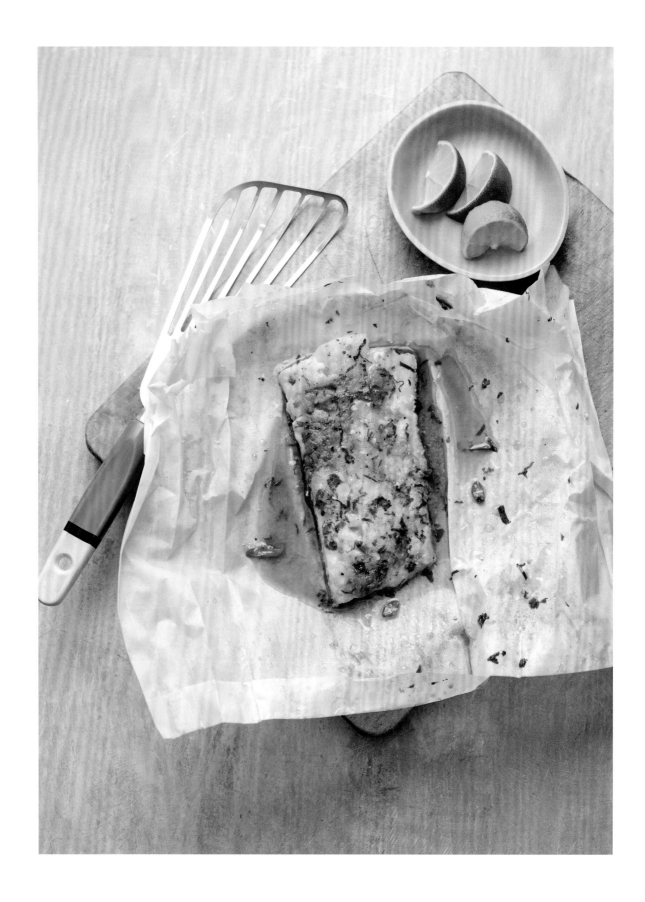

Cod in baking parchment

This recipe is a great one for preparing up to a couple of hours before required. This goes perfectly with my Broccoli, with spring onions, soy and chilli recipe on page 76. Once you have made this a few times, you can start experimenting with other fish, such as salmon, haddock, whiting and even scallops.

Nutrition notes

Cod is a lean protein source that's full of essential vitamins and minerals. Cod is high in B vitamins that have many essential functions in the body, such as helping to metabolize our food, releasing further nutrients and energy. Cod also provides the essential minerals of phosphorus and selenium. Phosphorus is an essential component of our bones and teeth, while selenium has a critical role in DNA synthesis. The fresh ginger in this recipe provides gingerol, a natural component of ginger root. Gingerol benefits gastrointestinal motility - the rate at which food exits the stomach and continues along the digestive tract. Eating ginger encourages efficient digestion.

Equipment | 2 x 30cm x 30cm (12in x 12in) pieces of aluminium foil | 20cm x 20cm (8in x 8in) piece of greaseproof paper | 40cm x 30cm (16in x 12in) oven tray

1 Preheat the oven to 180°C/400°F/gas mark 6.

2 Place a piece of the foil onto the oven tray followed by the greaseproof paper. Lay the cod fillets in the middle of the paper.

3 Using a fine microplane, grate the garlic and ginger into a bowl. Add the olive oil, soy sauce and lemon juice and mix well. Pour this mix over the cod. Place the other piece of foil on top and fold around the edges to seal and create a pouch.

4 When ready to cook, place in the centre of the oven and cook for 10–15 minutes. After this time, remove from the oven and leave to rest for 5 minutes before breaking the foil seal. Add the sliced chilli and coriander. Pour all the residual juices collected in the foil parcel over the fish to serve.

Serves 2

2 x 200g (7oz) skinless cod fillets
1 garlic clove
10g (¼oz) ginger
1 tablespoon extra virgin olive oil
1 teaspoon soy sauce
Juice of 1 lemon
1 red bird's eye chilli, finely sliced
5g (⅛oz) fresh coriander, finely chopped

Flaked mackerel with scrambled egg and cottage cheese

I have always loved hot smoked mackerel, and eating it flaked through scrambled eggs is delicious. I eat this on sourdough toast with a drizzle of extra virgin olive oil and a side order of kimchi. When buying your smoked mackerel, go for natural smoked that has not been coloured, as it makes a huge difference and is a lot better for you.

Nutrition notes

For a small fish, mackerel packs a nutrient punch. Mackerel is incredibly rich in nutrients, especially vitamin B12 (essential for red blood cell formation and a healthy central nervous system) and selenium (essential for reproduction, thyroid hormone metabolism, DNA synthesis and protection from oxidative damage and infection). Pound for pound, mackerel also contains some of the highest amounts of omega-3 polyunsaturated fatty acid (omega-3 PUFA). Historical studies have shown that communities that eat large quantities of fatty fish have lower incidence rates of cardiovascular disease. This is likely attributed to the omega-3 PUFAs, which when consumed in adequate amounts, can beneficially alter cholesterol and lower triglyceride levels in the blood.

Serves 2

Extra virgin olive oil
4 eggs, whisked
2 skinless hot smoked mackerel fillets, flaked
1 tablespoon chopped fresh chives
1 large shallot, finely diced
60g (2oz) cottage cheese
Flaked sea salt and freshly ground white pepper, to taste

1   Drizzle a little olive oil into a heavy-based saucepan and place on a medium heat. Crack in the eggs and slowly start to cook. Use a spatula to keep the mix moving and scrambling, until cooked to your liking.

2   Remove the pan from the heat and add the smoked mackerel, chives and shallots. Season with the salt and pepper, place a dollop of cottage cheese on top and serve.

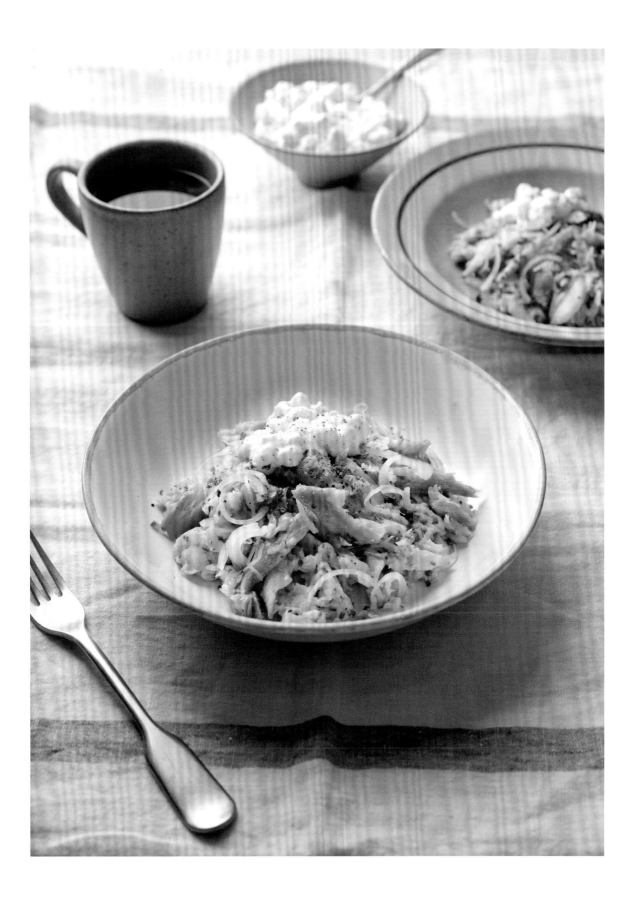

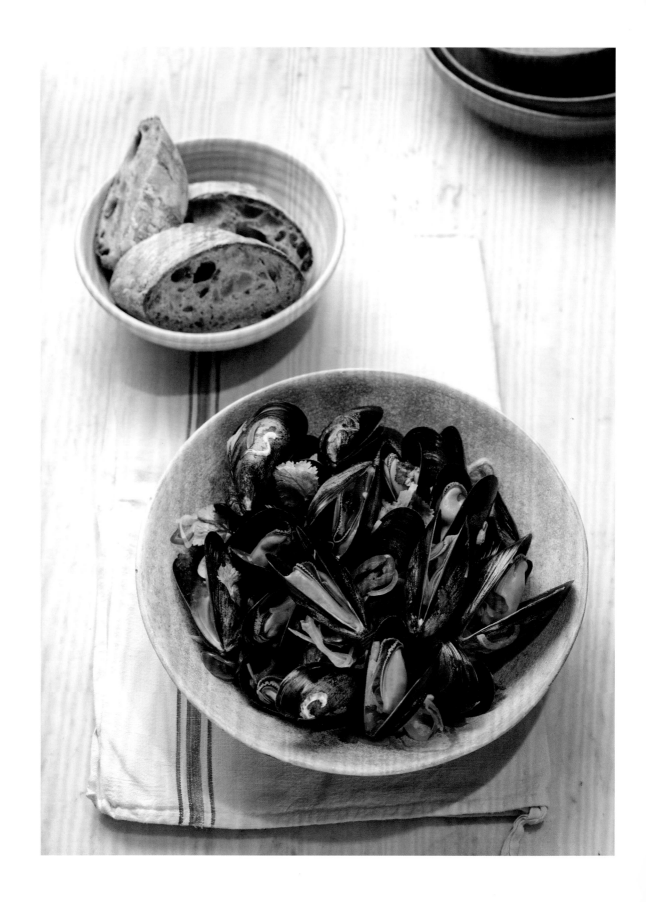

Mussels in white wine and coriander

With all shellfish there are a few house rules, and when it comes to mussels, if they stay open when tapped, or if they stay closed once cooked, they should be discarded. You can ask your fishmonger to clean mussels for you if you are not sure about this bit of prep, but if you are, give it a go, as it is not too difficult and you will learn a new skill. It is paramount also to not overcook the mussels, as they will turn into ping-pong balls, so as soon as they open, take them off the heat and they will be full, plump and juicy. You can also use dill, parsley or chives in this recipe, if you want to switch up the flavours. Serve with a side of crusty bread spread with salted butter to mop up all the juices.

Nutrition notes

All seafood, including shellfish, is high in protein and low in fat. Mussels offer levels of protein and iron that can challenge any red meat option on a menu. Protein and iron are fundamental to health, providing the building blocks of and delivering oxygen to the entire human body.

Mussels are also packed full of zinc, which is essential for a strong and well-functioning immune system, and omega-3 polyunsaturated fatty acids, which are essential for heart health, and brain and blood function. Mussels truly are a super healthy, super delicious food.

Serves 2

500g (1lb 2oz) mussels (my
    preference is River Exe)
175ml (6fl oz) white wine
1 large shallot, finely sliced
1 red chilli, finely sliced
Large handful of chopped
    fresh coriander, stalks
    and leaves

1   Tip the mussels into a colander and wash them in cold running water. Remove any barnacles on the shell using a knife. If the mussels have a beard, gently pull it out and discard. If any of the mussels are open, tap them on a solid surface – if they don't close, they are dead and should not be eaten. Rinse the mussels again in fresh cold water to remove any bits of shell or barnacle and drain.

2   Set a saucepan on a high heat and add the white wine, shallot and chilli. When the mixture comes to the boil, add the mussels and place the lid on the pan. Cook the mussels for 3–4 minutes, shaking the pan from time to time to ensure they cook evenly. They are cooked when the shells have opened.

3   Remove the pan from the heat, remove and discard any mussels that are still closed, and sprinkle over the chopped coriander. Divide the mussels and all the juice between 2 bowls.

Natural smoked haddock with preserved lemon and cumin

This technique is great for making sure the fish doesn't dry out, as fish can easily do that. Be careful when picking the smoked haddock and go for naturally smoked, as the others can contain a high level of salt and colourings.

⌣ Nutrition notes

Fresh white fish like haddock is high in protein, so it keeps us feeling full for longer. It's also a great source of vitamins B6 and B12, both of which have an essential role in red blood cell production. Red blood cells contain a protein called haemoglobin, which is responsible for delivering oxygen throughout our bodies. A deficiency of vitamin B12 can adversely affect this oxygen delivery and has been associated with an increased risk of blood clots.

Equipment | 2 x 30cm x 30cm (12in x 12in) pieces of aluminium foil | 20cm x 20cm (8in x 8in) piece of greaseproof paper | 40cm x 30cm (16in x 12in) oven tray

Serves 2

1 Preheat the oven to 160°C/350°F/gas mark 4.

2 Place a piece of foil onto the oven tray followed by the greaseproof paper. Lay the smoked haddock in the middle of the paper. Scatter over the cumin seeds and preserved lemon. Drizzle with olive oil and add a pinch of salt and pepper. Drizzle a tablespoon of water around the fish, then place the other piece of foil on top and fold around the edges to create a pouch. When ready to cook, place in the centre of the oven and cook for 10-15 minutes.

3 Remove from the oven and leave to rest for 5 minutes before breaking the seal of the pouch to serve.

2 x 200g (7oz) smoked haddock fillets
2 teaspoons toasted cumin seeds
20g (¾oz) diced preserved lemon, pips removed
Extra virgin olive oil, for drizzling
Flaked sea salt and freshly ground black pepper, to taste

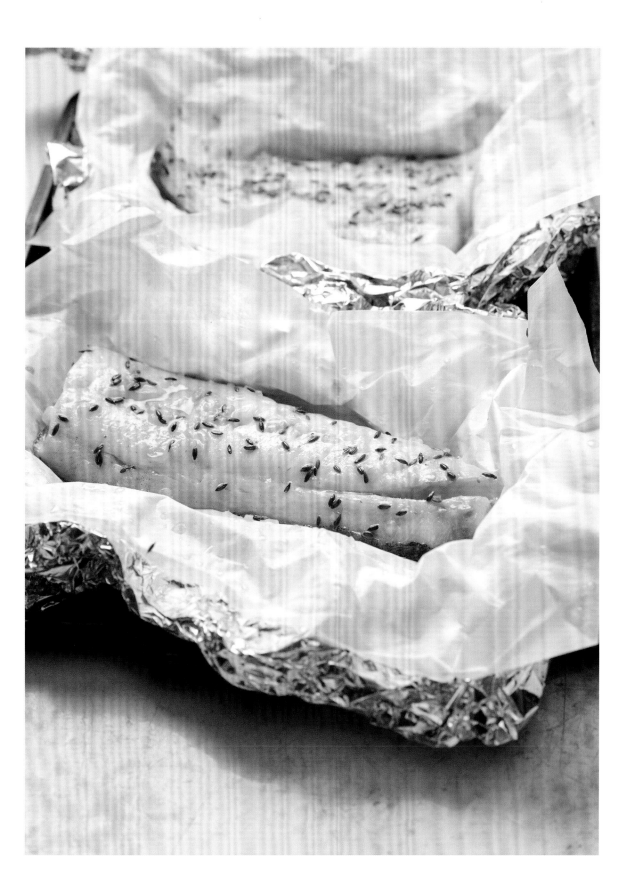

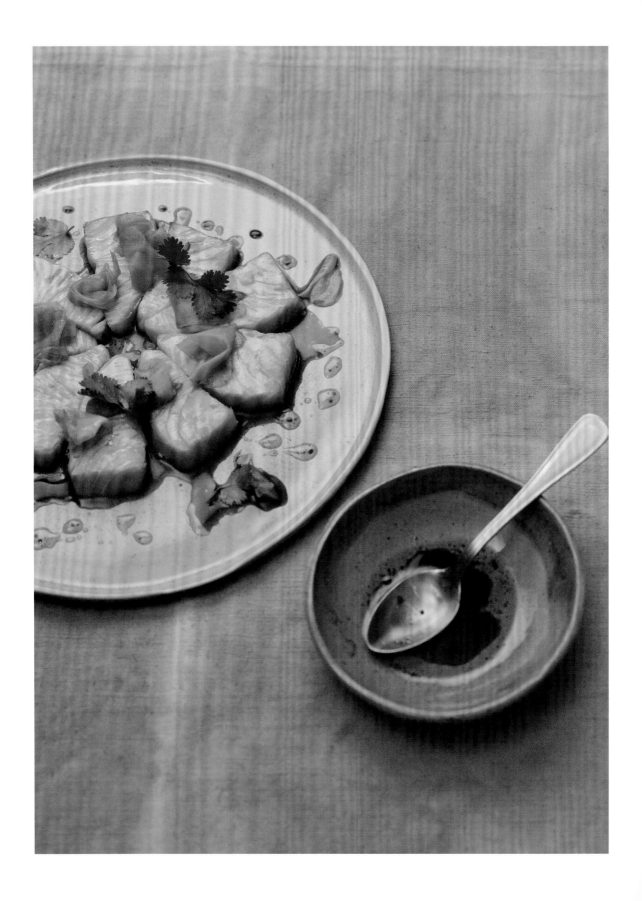

Warm grilled salmon with pickled ginger and soy sauce

The salmon is just barely cooked in this recipe, so make sure it is super fresh. The heat of the grill is enough to soften the fish, but make sure you don't overcook it, as it will dry out. You can buy pickled ginger from most supermarkets: find it in the Japanese section.

Nutrition notes

Salmon is a go-to ingredient for a diverse and heart-healthy diet. The consistent inclusion of oily fish alongside a diverse heart-healthy diet and regular exercise will have proven cardiovascular benefits. For more info on the health benefits of salmon, see page 104.

1   Preheat the grill to medium–high.

2   Slice the salmon into pieces around 2cm (¾in) thick. Place onto a flameproof plate and warm under the grill until lightly coloured – this should take about 1 minute; you want the fish to just lighten in colour a bit.

3   Make a dressing by combing a little olive oil, soy sauce and some of the juice from the ginger (this can be done to suit your own taste).

4   Remove the fish from the grill and spoon over the dressing. Add some of the chopped ginger and scatter over the coriander.

Serves 2

400g (14oz) organic salmon
   fillets (I like Loch Duart),
   scaled and pin-boned
Extra virgin olive oil, to taste
Soy sauce, to taste
Jarred natural sushi ginger,
   strained and chopped
   (reserve liquor for the
   dressing), to taste
10g (¼oz) chopped fresh
   coriander

Salmon XO

I love xo sauce: it is spicy, pungent and earthy, it goes well with all types of meat, fish and vegetables, and it is definitely worth the effort of making it because it lasts for a few months in the fridge. Dried scallops and dried shrimps are available online and from Chinese supermarkets, though you can buy good-quality xo sauces to use instead, but please be mindful of the salt and sugar content – that's why we make our own, so we can control every ingredient. Give it a go!

Nutrition notes

Once again in this recipe we are singing the praises of the heart-healthy omega-3 polyunsaturated fatty acid. We should remember that we should all aim to take a food-first approach to increasing our omega-3 content in our diet and oily fish such as salmon provides 15mg of omega-3 per gram of fish. An updated meta-analysis of 13 randomized controlled trials involving 127,477 participants concluded that omega-3 supplementation lowers risk for myocardial infarction, coronary heart disease and cardiovascular disease. Demonstrating excellent evidence to increase our omega-3 intake within our diets.

Equipment | Blender

1   Soak the dried scallops and shrimps in a bowl of water overnight in the fridge.

2   Blend the shiitake in a blender until coarse. Heat half the oil in a large heavy-based saucepan on a medium-high heat and cook the mushrooms for 10 minutes until caramelized. Blend the garlic, shallots and ginger in the same jug used for the mushrooms until coarse and add to the mushrooms, then cook for a further 10 minutes, until caramelized.

3   Add the chilli flakes and deglaze the pan with the sherry vinegar, Madeira and rice wine vinegar, scraping all the bits off the base of the pan. Cook for 20 minutes until the liquid has reduced to a thick glaze. Season with the soy and anchovy sauces to taste.

4   Blend the scallops and shrimp until coarse in a blender. In a separate pan, cook for 30 minutes in the remaining oil until caramelized.

5   Once cooked and caramelized, add it to the rest of the mix. Store in a sealed container in the fridge until ready to use.

Serves 2

100g (3½oz) dried scallops
25g (1oz) dried shrimps
250g (9oz) shiitake mushrooms
200ml (7fl oz) grapeseed oil
50g (2oz) garlic, peeled
250g (9oz) shallots, peeled
50g (2oz) ginger, peeled
5g (¼ teaspoon) chilli flakes
100g (3½oz) sherry vinegar
100g (3½oz) Madeira wine
50g (2oz) rice wine vinegar
Soy and anchovy sauce, to taste
2 x 200g (7oz) salmon fillets

6   To cook the fish, preheat the oven to 160°C/350°F/gas mark 4.

7   Lay the salmon fillets on a greaseproof-lined tray and spoon over 20g (¾oz) of the xo paste – you can add as much or as little as you like. Place in the oven and cook to your liking, around 10 minutes.

Sat's tip: Goes well with my Asian slaw on page 54.

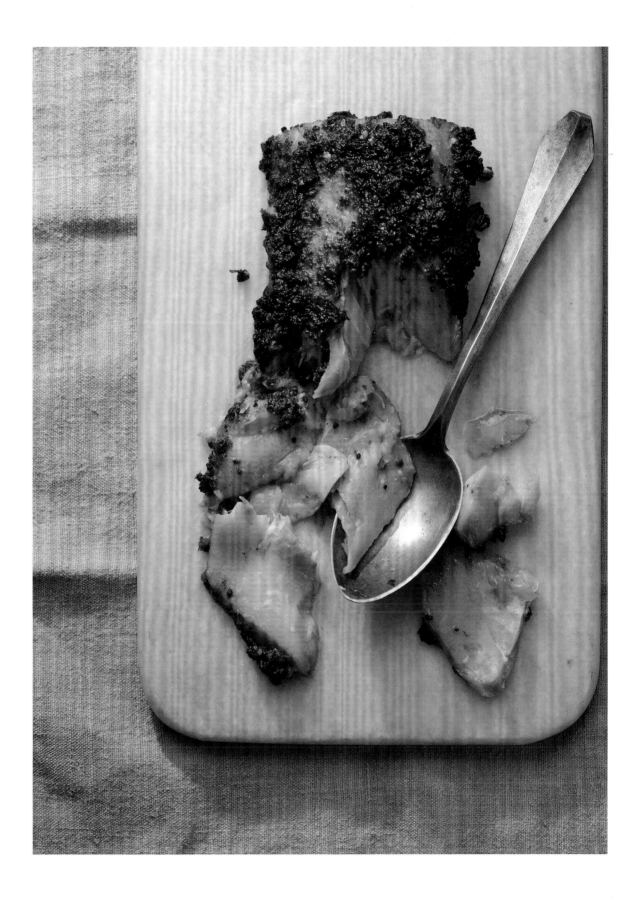

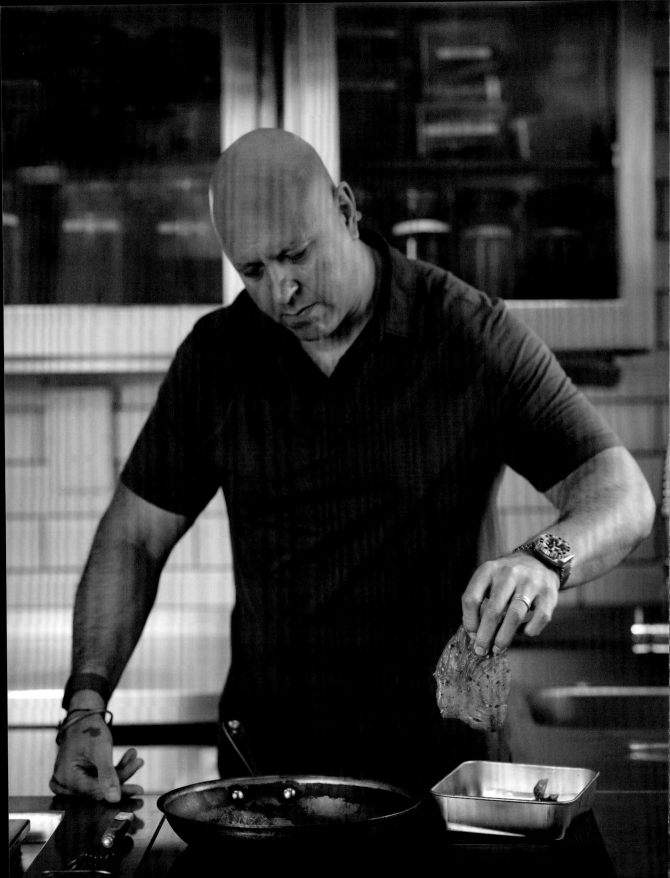

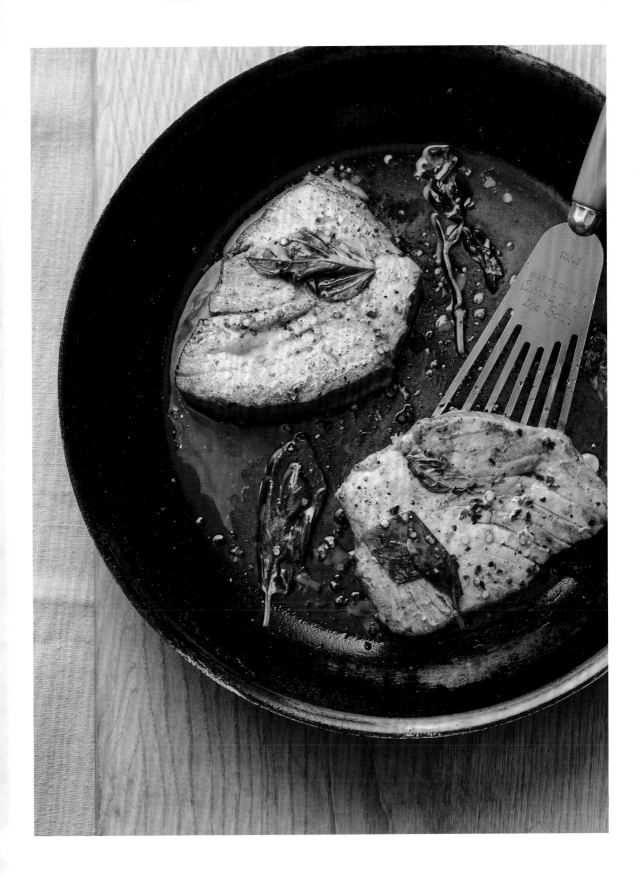

Pan-fried tuna marinated in soy, olive oil and basil

Make sure you use the freshest tuna you can get your hands on, as it will make all the difference. I sometimes replace the tuna with salmon, as it is rich in oils and lends itself to the flavours used here. Be careful not to overcook the fish, as it will dry out; remember you can serve super fresh fish slightly medium-rare.

Nutrition notes

Tuna has always been one of my favourite go-to post-exercise foods, because it is an excellent source of protein, which will aid muscle repair, and it makes us feel fuller for longer and keeps hunger pangs at bay. Plus it's packed with B vitamins (important for cell growth and brain function), and iron (essential for making red blood cells that carry oxygen around the body). Tuna is high in omega-3 fatty acids, and we should all try to increase the omega-3 content of our diet, as it can reduce triglycerides – a type of fat found in our blood – and so improves overall heart health.

1   Combine all the ingredients for the marinade in a shallow bowl. Add the tuna steaks, making sure they are well coated in the marinade. Leave in the fridge for 24 hours, turning a couple of times during this time.

2   When ready to cook, remove from the fridge and leave for 30 minutes. Remove the tuna from the marinade and place on kitchen paper to remove excess moisture.

3   Heat the sesame oil in a non-stick pan over a high heat, then add the tuna. Cook for 1-2 minutes on each side, depending on how you like it cooked. Remove from the pan and leave to rest for 2 minutes before serving.

Serves 2

400g (14oz) tuna loin cut
    into 2 'steaks'
10ml (¼fl oz) sesame oil

For the marinade
25g (1oz) basil, torn at the
    last minute
1 teaspoon chilli flakes
100ml (3½fl oz) extra
    virgin olive oil
25ml (1fl oz) soy sauce
Freshly ground black
    pepper, to taste

Cod with miso

Miso is a beautiful fermented paste made from rice, barley and soya beans that's used extensively in Japanese cuisine. I use it a lot at the restaurant and we even make a delicious salty fudge with it, but it really lends itself to fish, especially cod.

You can buy it from most supermarkets but I would try to source some really good-quality paste either online or from a Japanese supplier, as it is worth the effort.

Nutrition notes

Miso paste is essentially soya beans that have been fermented with koji. What is koji? It is a mould (*Aspergillus*) that has been cultivated from rice; over weeks or sometimes even years, the enzymes in the koji work to break down the structure of the soya beans into amino acids, fatty acids and simple sugars. Traditional Japanese cuisine uses the process of bean fermentation, which produces beneficial probiotic bacteria that, if they can survive the cooking process and transit to the gut, can have beneficial health effects.

Serves 2

2 x 200g (7oz) skinless cod fillets
75g (3oz) white miso paste
15g (½oz) sesame oil
15g (½oz) soy sauce
Juice of 1 lime

1 Preheat the oven to 180°C/400°F/gas mark 6.

2 Bring your cod out of the fridge 30 minutes before cooking, so that it can reach room temperature, then set on a baking tray.

3 In a bowl combine the miso paste, sesame oil, soy sauce and half the lime juice to a smooth paste. Divide the mix in half and spread over the 2 cod fillets. Place on a non-stick tray in the oven and cook for 10–15 minutes. Remove and leave to rest for a few minutes.

4 Once rested, squeeze over the remaining lime juice.

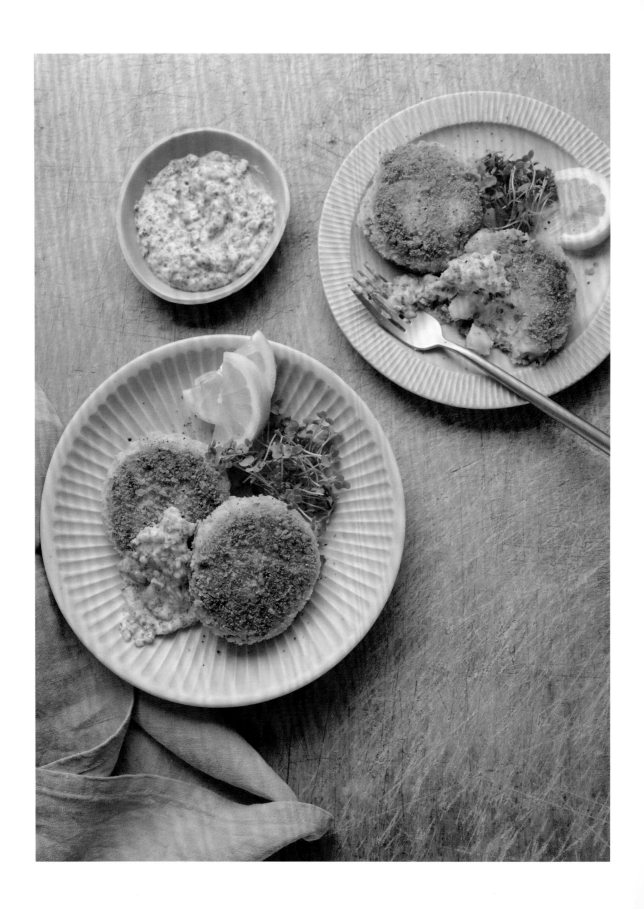

Sat's 'fishcakes'

Remember, we are only sealing the fishcakes and colouring them, not cooking them fully, as they will be completely cooked in the oven. Buying natural smoked cod means no artificial additives are added.

Nutrition notes

Although not as high as oily fish (salmon and mackerel), cod still provides a source of omega-3 polyunsaturated fatty acids, which are heart-healthy fatty acids thanks to their ability to reduce inflammation and bad LDL cholesterol levels in the blood. Cod also contains a high amount of phosphorus – roughly 20 per cent of our recommended daily intake can be obtained from this dish – and it is important for the health of our bones and teeth. It is also an excellent source of selenium, with roughly 40 per cent of our recommended daily intake coming from this dish, which is essential for making and protecting our DNA. So it really does help to make you, you!

Serves 2

300ml (10fl oz) milk

250g (9oz) natural smoked cod

400g (14oz) red potatoes peeled, boiled and drained as you would make mash (kept warm)

15g (½oz) chopped parsley

3 large organic eggs, whisked

Olive oil, for frying

Flaked sea salt and freshly ground black pepper, to taste

For the coating

300g (10oz) panko breadcrumbs

Zest of 1 lemon

2 large organic eggs, whisked

1 Pour the milk into a pan, season and gently bring to a very light simmer, then remove from the heat. Add the smoked cod to the hot milk, put the lid on and leave to poach. When cool enough to handle, flake the cooked cod into a bowl, add the warm potatoes and parsley and gently mix together.

2 Add the eggs and mix everything together, season with salt and pepper. Mould your fishcake mix into 6 equal balls and press down gently to slightly flatten, then refrigerate for at least 1 hour or until firm enough to handle.

3 Mix the lemon zest and panko breadcrumbs in one bowl and the egg wash in a separate bowl. Dip each fishcake into the egg until well coated, then shake off the excess and then dip into the breadcrumbs until evenly coated. Chill again for at least 20 minutes.

4 Preheat the oven to 180°C/350°F/gas mark 4.

5 Heat a splash of oil in a large frying pan over a medium heat. Cook each fishcake until the breadcrumbs have turned golden brown, then turn and repeat. You will need to do these 2 or 3 at a time to not overcrowd the pan.

6 Once browned, place them all on greaseproof paper on an oven tray and place in the oven for about 10 minutes. Remove from the oven and let cool slightly before you eat.

Scallops cooked over open coals

This recipe is all about the freshest scallops you can get your hands on. Using the shells as a baking tray on the open coals is a great way to cook them and save on washing up, and the odd spill of oil onto the coals and flare up all adds flavour to the finished dish. Once cooked the scallops need to be eaten quickly to get them at their best, so make sure you are ready to eat as soon as they are cooked. You will notice there is no salt in this recipe, and that is because the soy is more than enough.

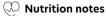 **Nutrition notes**

Scallops have a very impressive pound-for-pound nutritional content. They are a high-quality lean protein source and are full of heart-healthy omega-3 polyunsaturated fatty acids. For more info on omega-3 polyunsaturated fatty acids, see page 111. Scallops are an excellent source of trace minerals, including copper, selenium and zinc. These trace minerals, although required in very small quantities, can be deficient in some diets. Adequate zinc and selenium are important for a healthy immune system, and there is some evidence to suggest copper deficiency may increase the risk of heart disease. Therefore, these little shellfish can be a great heart-healthy nutritional treat.

Equipment | Charcoal barbecue

1 Light your barbecue at least 30 minutes before it is needed, with the griddle plate removed.

2 In a medium bowl add the sesame oil, garlic, ginger, soy sauce and pepper and mix well.

3 Lay out all your scallop shells and divide the dressing mix equally between the shells. Now add the scallops on top and carefully place the shells directly on the barbecue coals - make sure you use an oven mitt for this. The scallops won't take long to start simmering in the dressing, so be quick to take them off as they will cook in 3-4 minutes.

Serves 2

8 super fresh scallops, removed from shells and shells washed and cleaned

For the dressing

5ml (1 teaspoon) sesame oil

10g (¼oz) garlic, grated

10g (¼oz) ginger, grated

15ml (1 tablespoon) soy sauce

Freshly ground black pepper

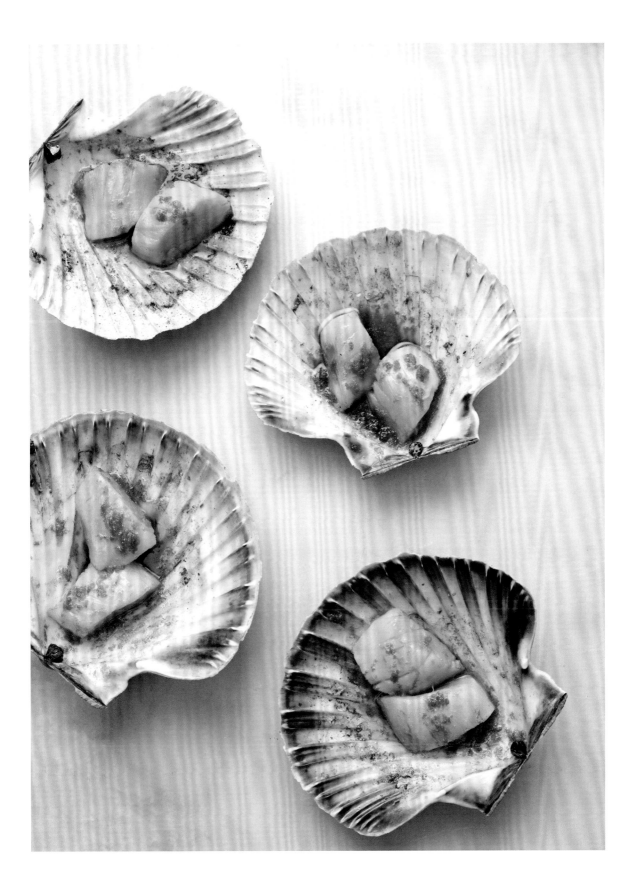

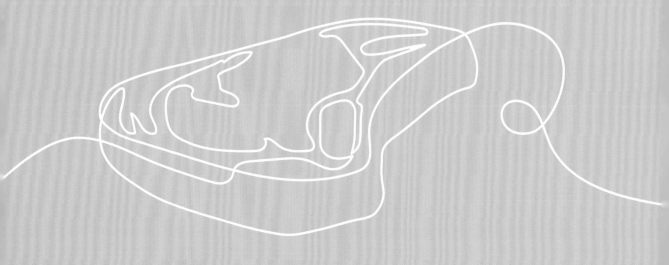

5

meat

Spatchcock chicken with roasted roots and herbs

I would eat this every day of the week if I had my way, as it has everything for me. The chicken is laid out so it cooks quicker and more evenly, and there are always leftovers, which is my favourite part. Add some shredded chicken to a Potato flatbread (page 162) with a dollop of Hummus (page 165) – heaven.

Nutrition notes

Chicken is a common dietary staple and one of the most popular types of meat to eat. Although not normally considered a health food, diversity is key and chicken is a valuable component to any diet. Chicken is lean and high in protein, and diets high in protein can increase our feelings of fullness and help us to maintain muscle mass. Maintaining a high-protein intake is especially important as we age, because it can help minimize age-related muscle loss, which is a risk factor for falls and reduced quality of life.

1   Preheat the oven to 160°C/350°F/gas mark 4.

2   Wash your root veg but don't peel them, instead leave them whole or chopped up – the choice is yours. Place the vegetables in a mixing bowl, add the thyme and oregano, season with salt and pepper and drizzle with olive oil. Halve or crush the garlic bulb and mix into the veg. Lay out on a roasting tray and place the chicken on top. Season the chicken with salt and pepper and cook in the oven for 1 hour.

3   Remove from the oven and leave to rest for 30 minutes. Remove the crushed garlic bulb and smother it over the bird before serving.

Serves 2

A selection of your
   favourite root
   vegetables
25g (1oz) thyme leaves
15g (½oz) oregano leaves
Extra virgin olive oil
1 bulb of garlic
1 medium chicken,
   spatchcocked (ask your
   butcher to do this)
Flaked sea salt and freshly
   ground black pepper, to
   taste

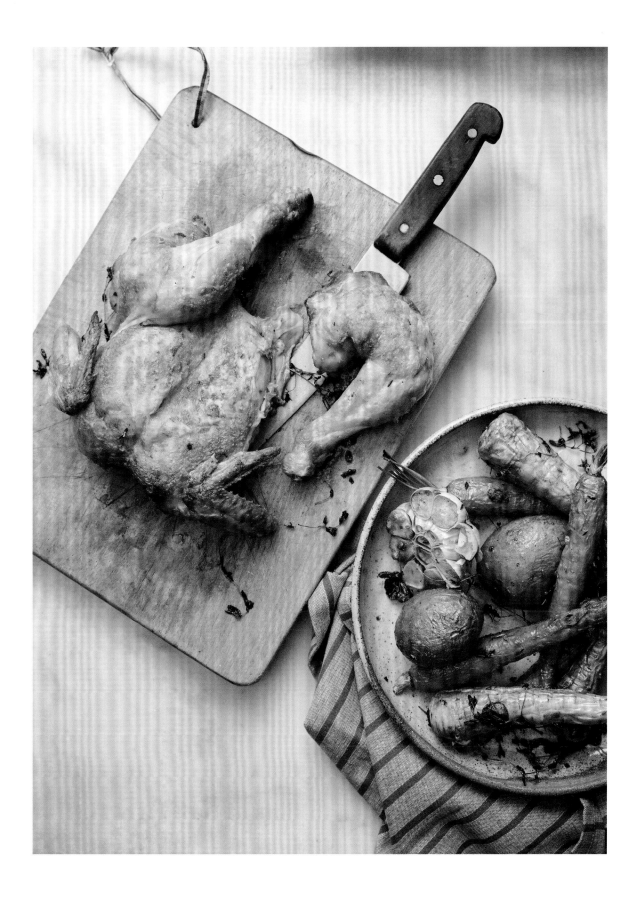

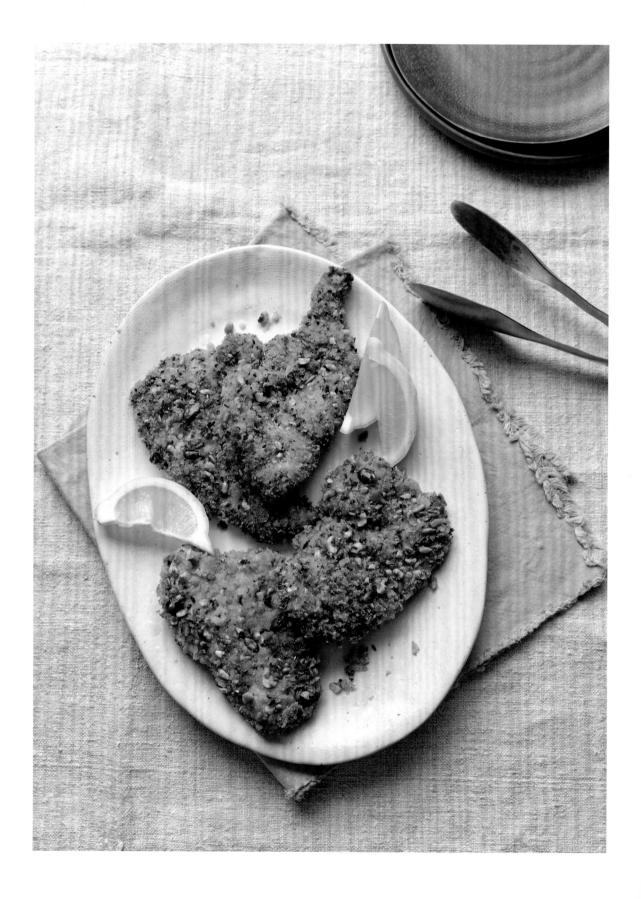

Nut and seed crispy chicken escalope

I love this mix for my chicken escalope; I make more than I need and use what I need for however many chicken breasts I am using and save the rest in a freezer bag or an airtight container in the cupboard, where it will last for several weeks. The seeded mix adds an incredible texture to the chicken and it is definitely something you will come back to again and again.

Nutrition notes

Nuts are very energy dense – most contain 50–60 per cent fat – so in the past they were incorrectly considered unhealthy. This high fat content, though, is mainly unsaturated healthy fat like oleic acid (similar to that found in olive oil) and either poly- or monounsaturated fat. Nuts are also high in protein (10–30 per cent) as well as in heart- and gut-healthy fibre (5 per cent). A large long-term clinical trial showed that men and women over the age of 60 consuming 30g of nuts per week had 30 per cent less risk of heart disease and stroke over a five-year follow-up compared to a group on a low-fat diet. In a nutshell, nuts are a great source of unsaturated fats, fibre and protein and we should all aim to consume a good mix of unprocessed nuts and seeds every week.

Equipment | Air fryer

1. Combine all the crumb coating ingredients in a bowl and spread some of the crumb coating over a plate (store the rest for another time). In another bowl, whisk the eggs with the harissa and some salt and pepper.

2. Place the chicken in the egg wash, making sure it's coated all over, then shake off any excess and press the chicken into the crumb coating, making sure it is completely covered. Set aside for 30 minutes.

3. Preheat your air fryer to 190°C/375°F. Place the chicken breasts on a piece of foil, spray with oil, then add them to the air fryer and cook for 8 minutes. Once cooked, rest for 2 minutes and then serve.

Serves 2

2 eggs
1 teaspoon dried harissa powder
2 chicken breasts, cut in half and slightly flattened
Extra virgin olive oil spray

For the crumb coating
100g (3½oz) panko breadcrumbs
1 tablespoon toasted cumin seeds, crushed
1 tablespoon toasted coriander seeds, crushed

1 tablespoon pumpkin seeds
1 tablespoon sunflower seeds
1 tablespoon chia seeds
1 tablespoon poppy seeds
1 tablespoon black sesame seeds
50g (2oz) pine nuts, chopped
50g (2oz) nibbed almonds
Pinch each of flaked sea salt and freshly ground black pepper

Minced chicken burger with ginger, garlic and baharat

This is a great alternative to a beef burger, delicious and nutritional. It is important you get your butcher to mince the chicken for you for this recipe, as breast meat is very lean, but you do need some fat to create a juicy burger, which is why we add the thigh meat. Baharat is a spice mixture or blend used in Middle Eastern cuisines that's available in most supermarkets. You can cook this on the barbecue, too, but be careful not to dry out the meat.

Serves 2

200g (7oz) chicken breast mince
100g (3½oz) chicken thigh mince
1 large shallot, finely diced
10g (¼oz) minced garlic
10g (½oz) grated ginger
1 teaspoon baharat spice
Flaked sea salt, to taste
Extra virgin olive oil, for frying

1   Mix together the chicken minces, shallot, garlic, ginger and baharat. Season with a pinch of salt and form the mix into 4 equal-sized balls.

2   Place a large non-stick frying pan over a high heat and drizzle in a little olive oil. Add the chicken balls and push each one down using the back of a spatula to flatten into patties. Cook for 4 minutes on each side – the 'burgers' should be golden brown and cooked through.

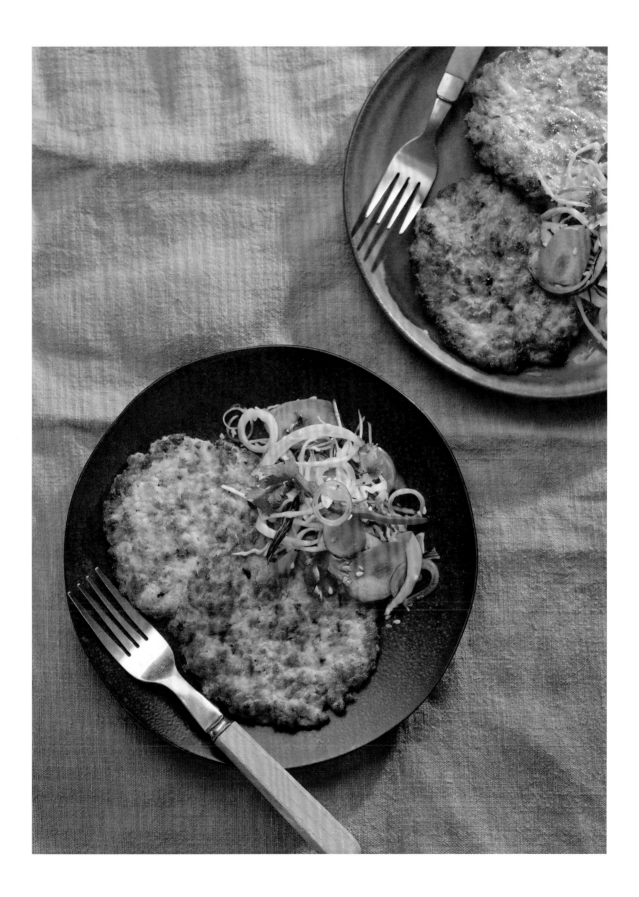

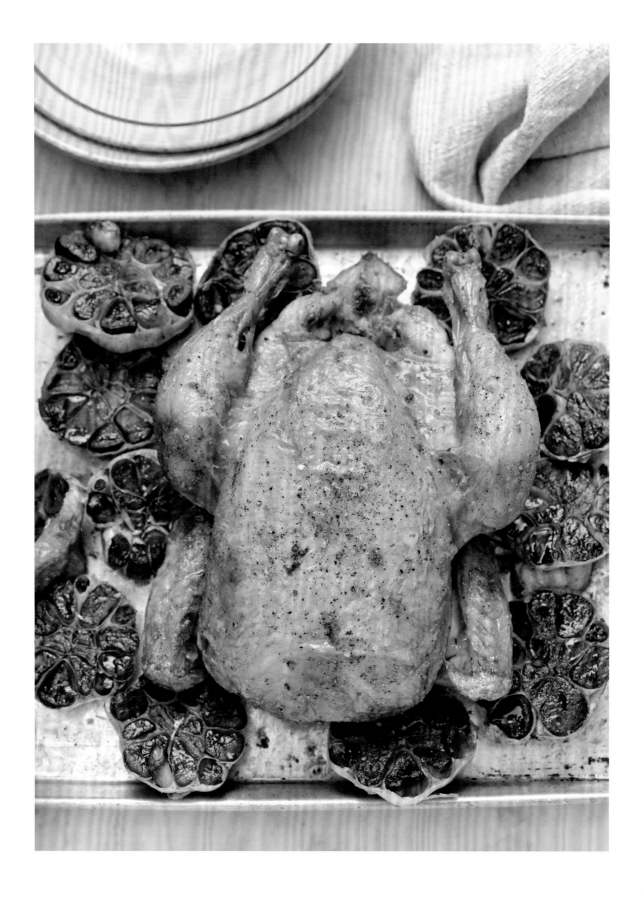

Chicken with seven bulbs of garlic

Yes, I know, this sounds excessive but I love garlic, and I can eat roasted garlic all day. This is a brilliant way to allow the cooking juices and garlic to caramelize on the bottom of the roasting tin to create an incredible flavour. Each clove just pops out and you can eat them like that or collect them all, add the cooking liquors and make a paste, which can then be spread all over the chicken and eaten.

Nutrition notes

Seven bulbs of garlic will not only keep a herd of hungry vampires away, but it's also great for our health. Garlic is one of the oldest cultivated plants, with a long history of purported medicinal effects. The research is now starting to catch up and provide supporting evidence for its historical medicinal use. Garlic has an impressive array of bioactive compounds, including phenolic compounds, organic sulfides, saponins and polysaccharides. Many risk factors for cardiovascular disease (obesity, high blood pressure, insulin resistance and high serum triglycerides levels) may be modified by some of garlic's compounds.

Serves 2

7 bulbs of garlic, cut in half,
   widthways, skin on
1 x 2kg (4lb 8oz) cornfed chicken
Extra virgin olive oil
Flaked sea salt and freshly
   ground black pepper, to taste

1   Preheat the oven to 160°C/350°F/gas mark 4.

2   Take a roasting tray big enough to fit the garlic and lay the bulbs cut-side down. Sit the chicken on top and drizzle with olive oil. Season with salt and pepper then place in the oven and cook through for 1 hour and 45 minutes – the juices should run clear when you pierce the thigh with a skewer.

3   Remove from the oven, cover with foil and leave to rest for 20 minutes.

Chicken meatballs with butter beans and lemon

Chicken meatballs make an amazing change to the usual beef or pork. This recipe is Italian-inspired and the butter bean stew that accompanies the meatballs is delicious and wholesome. The lemon here adds some great acidity and the anchovies a big hit of umami. Make sure you get the best-quality chicken for this - I get the butcher to mince 300g (10oz) of breast meat and 100g (3½oz) of skinned and boned thigh meat for me, which adds some fat - or the meatballs can become dry.

⌣ **Nutrition notes**

Like other legumes, butter beans contain phytosterols, which include plant sterols and stanols and are present in small quantities. Structurally similar to cholesterol, these phytosterols can compete with cholesterol for absorption by your digestive system. When your body digests plant sterols instead of cholesterol, it removes some of the cholesterol as waste, resulting in lowered cholesterol levels. Butter beans also provide extra protein to this recipe, and these little legumes are also a great fibre and nutrient source, supporting healthy weight loss, enhanced blood sugar control and improved heart health.

1 Combine all the ingredients for the meatballs, except the olive oil. Divide the mix into 24 and roll into balls, placing them on a piece of greaseproof paper.

2 Heat a large pan over a medium-high heat. Add a splash of olive oil and fry off the meatballs for a few minutes, making sure they are nicely browned all over. Add the beans, tomatoes and chicken stock to the pan, bring to a gentle simmer and leave to cook for 1½ hours. Give it a stir every now and again to make sure the meatballs are not sticking.

3 When finished, season if needed and add a drizzle of olive oil. Serve scattered with the reserved parsley and the pine nuts.

Serves 2

For the meatballs

400g (14oz) chicken mince
Zest of 1 lemon
5g (⅛oz) chopped parsley, plus 5g (⅛oz) extra for garnish
50g (2oz) Parmesan, grated
25g (1oz) fine fresh breadcrumbs
2 garlic cloves, grated
4 anchovy fillets (I use Ortiz)
20g (¾oz) basil, chopped
Pinch of flaked sea salt and freshly ground black pepper
Olive oil, for frying and drizzling

For the stew

2 x 400g (14oz) tins of butter beans, drained
1 x 400g (14oz) tin of chopped tomatoes
250ml (9fl oz) chicken stock
20g (¾oz) pine nuts, to serve

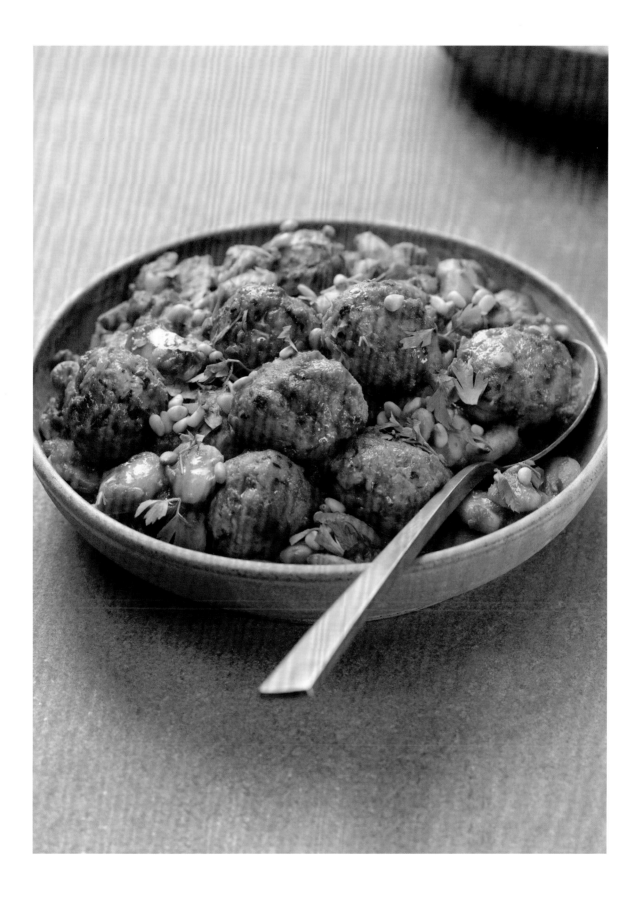

Dry-fried spiced lamb mince

I like this recipe for its speed, as I can knock it up in 20 minutes or so. Some helpful tips are to pre-mix your spices in an airtight container, in a dark cupboard, for up to three months, so you just need to add one spoon or so rather than having to weigh them all out separately and mix them up. Having said that, always purchase spices in small quantities as they will better retain their freshness. The best lettuce for this is anything that creates a cup-like shell for you to fill – almost like a taco shell.

1   Heat the oil in a large non-stick frying pan over a high heat. Add the lamb and cook until golden brown and crispy, then drain off some of the fat.

2   Add the wet mix and cook for 5 minutes, then add the dry mix and cook for a further 3 minutes. Pour in the water, cook for 2 minutes and remove from the heat.

3   On 2 large serving plates, cover the base with the lettuce leaves. Scatter the lamb mix over the lettuce and top with the yoghurt and pomegranate seeds. To finish, scatter over the mint and coriander leaves.

Serves 2

Extra virgin olive oil
400g (14oz) lean lamb mince
75ml (3oz) water
2 baby gem lettuces, leaves separated and washed
50g (2oz) natural yoghurt
30g (1oz) pomegranate seeds
5g (⅛oz) coriander leaves, chopped
5g (⅛oz) mint leaves, chopped

For the wet mix
1 large shallot, finely sliced
15g (½oz) grated ginger
15g (½oz) grated garlic
1 bird's eye chillies, finely sliced

For the dry mix
1 teaspoon ground cinnamon
1 teaspoon ground cumin
1 teaspoon ground coriander
1 teaspoon ras el hanout

Lamb chops with harissa

This recipe blows my mind because it is the easiest thing in the world - you just need a freezer bag, a jar of harissa and some olive oil, then seal and shake the bag and leave to chill for 3-4 hours. When you cook this, make sure you include some gnarly caramelized, charred bits, as they really add flavour. Make sure you ask your butcher to French trim the lamb chops for you, unless you are confident in doing this. I eat these like a lollipop, with mint yoghurt and a lemon wedge and with Potato flatbread (page 162) and my Raw cauliflower salad (page 53) on the side.

Nutrition notes

With ageing our body's ability to repair and build muscle tissue is reduced, and therefore we should ensure we eat plenty of lean protein sources to support muscle repair. This can support healthy ageing and potentially reduce the onset of frailty and risk of falls. Lamb can be an excellent lean protein source, supporting our intake of our essential amino acids within a diverse diet. There are nine essential amino acids (including isoleucine, leucine and valine), which are termed essential and which we must obtain from our diet. These are necessary for supporting muscle tissue growth and repair, amongst many other functions in the body - including supporting the making of hormones and neurotransmitters, supporting the immune and digestive systems).

Equipment | 1 large sealable freezer bag | Barbecue

1   Place the harissa and olive oil in the freezer bag, add the lamb chops, seal and massage to coat the lamb. Transfer to the fridge to marinate for 3 hours.

2   Get your barbecue ready when you take the lamb out of the fridge; this will allow the lamb to come up to temperature while the barbecue is heating up. Remove the chops from the bag and cook for 4-5 minutes on each side.

3   Remove from the heat and drizzle with more olive oil and the lemon juice, and scatter over the lemon zest and torn mint.

Serves 2

75g (3oz) rose harissa
    (I like Belazu)
25g (1oz) extra virgin olive
    oil, plus extra to serve
6 lamb chops, French
    trimmed (see intro)
Zest and juice of 1 lemon
Small handful of mint
    leaves, torn

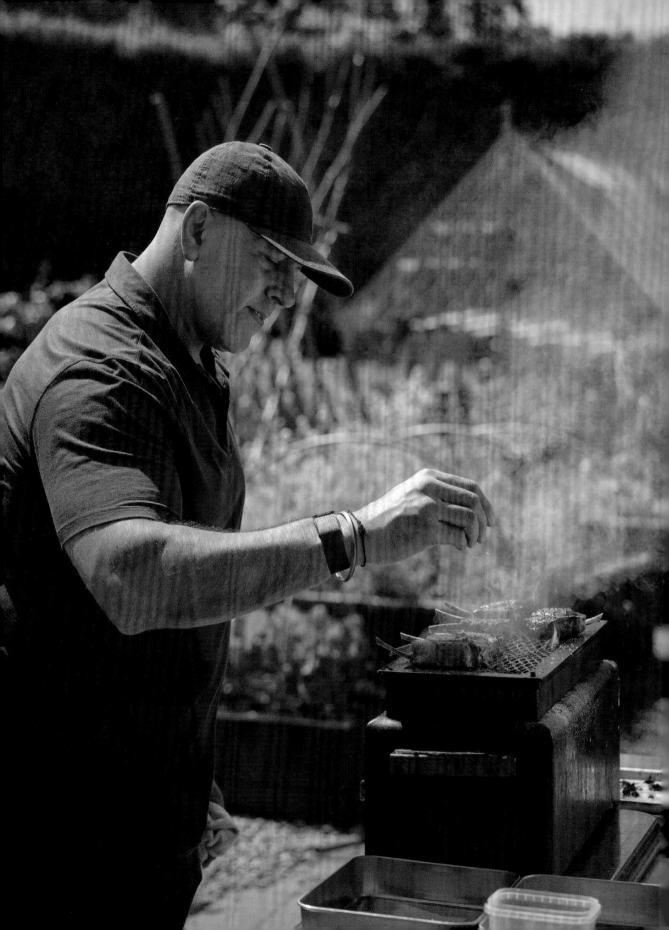

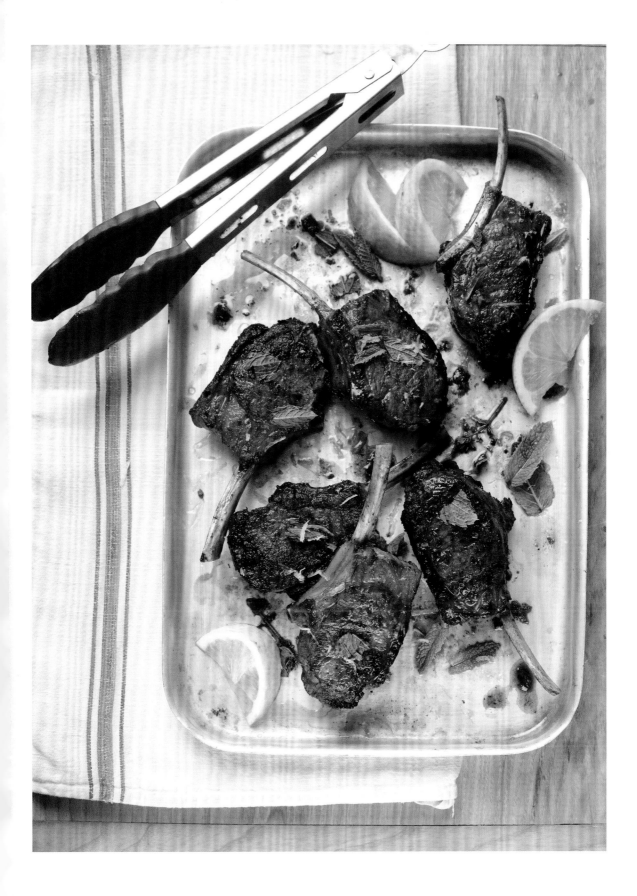

My flattened lamb kofta/kebab

I make this nearly every other week when it is barbecue season, or at least once a month when it isn't. You can make a batch of the mince and flatten it out and freeze it in between layers of baking parchment and it only takes minutes to defrost, or you can even cook from frozen as it is so thin. I serve this with flatbreads and Greek yoghurt.

🧠 **Nutrition notes**

Lamb meat is a high-quality protein source that is packed with all nine of the body's essential amino acids to support growth and maintenance. It therefore provides an optimal choice whenever muscle tissue needs to be built or repaired. Lamb not only helps preserve muscle mass but may also be important for muscle function. This is because it contains another amino acid called beta-alanine, which your body uses to produce carnosine, a substance necessary for muscle function.

Serves 2

400g (14oz) 10%-fat lamb mince
1 teaspoon ground cumin
1 teaspoon ground coriander
1 teaspoon chilli flakes
1 teaspoon grated ginger
1 teaspoon minced garlic
1 teaspoon ras el hanout
1 teaspoon dried harissa
Pinch each of flaked sea salt and freshly ground black pepper

1   Place all the ingredients in a bowl and mix well. Cover and leave to rest in the fridge for a minimum of 2 hours.

2   Divide the mix into 4 balls, then place each ball between 2 sheets of greaseproof paper and roll out to a thickness of 1cm (½in).

3   Place a non-stick frying pan on a high heat and sear the lamb sheets for 1 minute on each side. You are dry frying, so be careful not to burn it, you want it only slightly charred. Remove the lamb from the pan and serve.

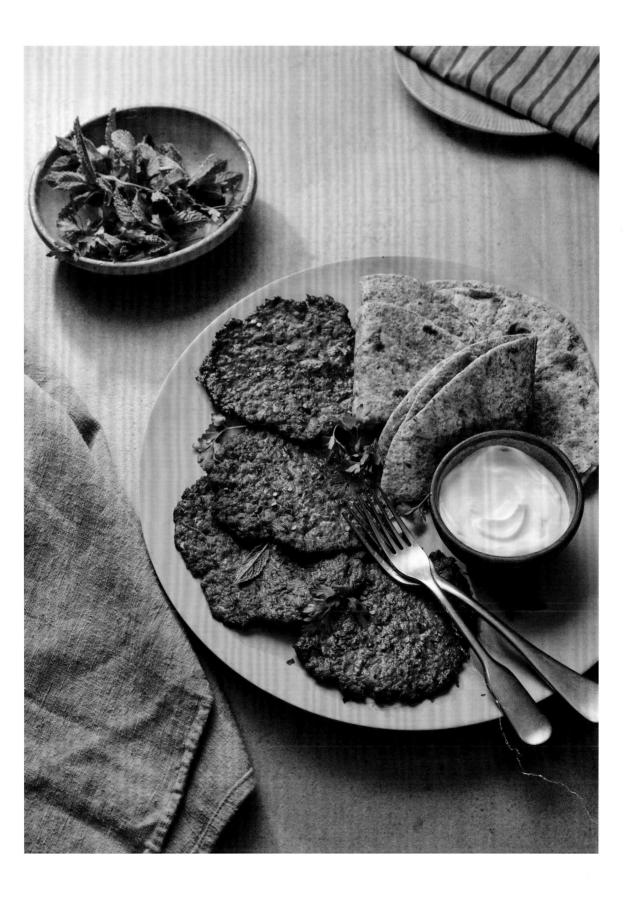

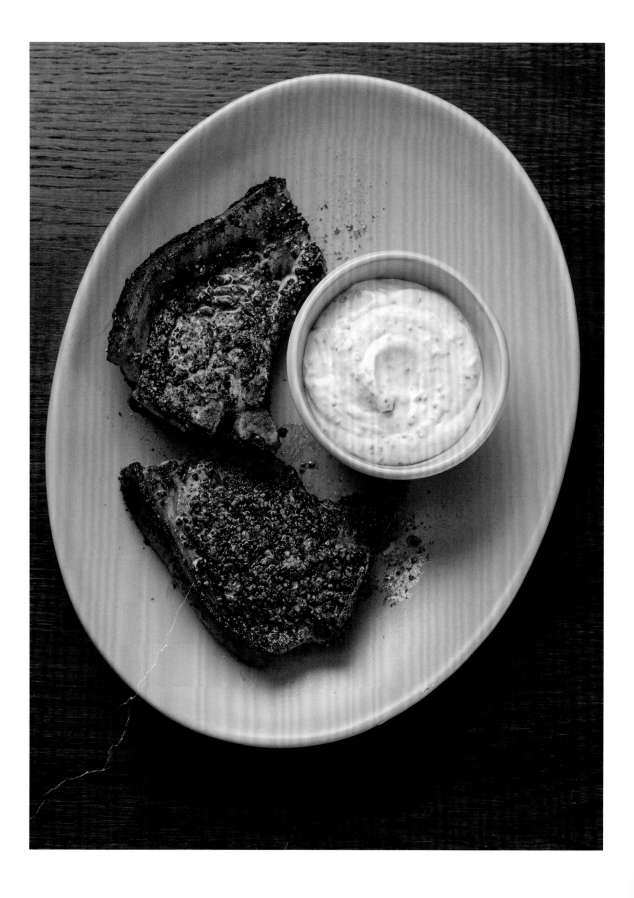

Peppered pork chop with mustards

Adding peppercorns gives a great level of heat to the dish and gives the meat a nice crust when cooking - be sure to buy the best free-range pork you can to make sure the flavour is intense. With pork you need a level of fat on it, so trim it only if it is excessive. The meat should have a beautiful golden colour and deep crust when cooked. The triple mustard crème fraîche adds a cool, sharp flavour, and it can be used with steak and chicken dishes as well.

Nutrition notes

Lean pork can be an excellent addition to a balanced healthy diet. High in protein and rich in many minerals and vitamins, pork contains all nine essential amino acids which are necessary to support the growth and maintenance of healthy muscles and bones. Plus, as with many lean meat sources, it delivers key nutrients such as thiamine, niacin, vitamin B12 and zinc. Some studies have linked thiamine deficiency with an increased risk of heart failure.

Serves 2

2 x 350g (12oz) pork chops
2 tablespoons black peppercorns, crushed in a pestle and mortar to a coarse grain
Flaked sea salt
30ml (1fl oz) extra virgin olive oil

Triple mustard crème fraîche
1 teaspoon wholegrain mustard
½ teaspoon Dijon mustard
½ teaspoon English mustard
100g (3½oz) crème fraîche

1 First make the triple mustard crème fraîche; fold the mustards into the crème fraîche in a bowl, cover and set aside in the fridge.

2 Encrust the pork chop in the peppercorns and some salt. Heat the oil in a heavy-based pan on a medium-high heat, then add the seasoned pork. Lower to a medium heat and cook for 10-15 minutes, turning the pork every minute. When cooked, remove from the pan to a plate and let the meat rest for 10 minutes before serving, along with the triple mustard crème fraîche.

Chunky venison chilli with bitter chocolate

This recipe is a really good way to get some game into your menu. I love game and eat it a lot, because it is a lean and healthy meat, and is low in cholesterol too. The spicing in this recipe is all about getting that balance of bitter chocolate with the kick of heat from the chilli - a perfect combo.

Nutrition notes

Venison is an excellent choice when you need a meaty hit for a recipe but want a leaner choice compared to other red meat. Although there is cholesterol in venison, the amount is not significantly greater than other red meat, but venison is lower in fat and saturated fat so it can be used in moderation in diverse heart-healthy diet. It also provides a lean protein source, helping provide essential amino acids and keeping you full for longer.

1   Heat a large heavy-based pan on a medium-high heat. When hot, add the olive oil, then add the venison and seal the meat until nice and evenly browned. Season with salt and pepper.

2   Now add the wet mix and sweat the vegetables until soft, 5–6 minutes.

3   Then add the dry mix and cook out for about 5 minutes, stirring occasionally to keep the mixture moving in the pan.

4   Add the tomato paste and cook out for 2–3 minutes, then pour in the stock and kidney beans, cover and cook gently over a low-medium heat for about 2 hours or until the meat is tender.

5   Once cooked, taste for seasoning and grate the chocolate into the chilli - this will make the dish rich and unctuous with a deep level of spice. You can serve this with my Potato flatbread (page 162) or my Raw cauliflower salad (page 53).

Serves 2

75ml (3oz) olive oil
400g (14oz) venison haunch, cut into 4cm (1½in) chunks
1 tablespoon tomato paste
400ml (14fl oz) chicken or beef stock
1 x 400g (14oz) tin of kidney beans, drained
75g (3oz) dark chocolate (80% cocoa solids)
Flaked sea salt and freshly ground black pepper, to taste

For the wet mix
2 medium white onions, chopped into 1cm (½in) dice
2 red chillies, thinly sliced
4 celery sticks, chopped into 1cm (½in) dice
1 leek, chopped into 1cm (½in) dice
1 sprig of thyme
2 bay leaves

For the dry mix
1 cinnamon stick
1 teaspoon bitter cocoa powder
2 teaspoons chilli powder
1 teaspoon flaked chillies
1 teaspoon smoked paprika
1 teaspoon ground cumin

Minced venison and oyster mushroom winter warmer

This is a great, warming dish for a cold winters day and when you don't have a lot of time on your hands. Full of heady spices and heat from the chillies, this is a quick dish to prepare, and the textures of the mushrooms and the spicy venison are a brilliant contrast to eat.

When you fry the mince, don't be alarmed by the meat sticking to the bottom of the pan, as the browning of the meat adds a depth of flavour, but be careful not to scorch it. When you add the dry mix, everything will stick but adding the wet mix will help lift all the stuck particles as the moisture is released, leaving an almost clean pan again - this is a little chef's tip called deglazing.

1   Heat a large heavy-based pan or wok on a medium-high heat. When hot, add the olive oil, then add the venison mince and fry until golden and separated.

2   Add the mushrooms and butter to the pan and cook for 10-12 minutes, until the mushrooms are golden-brown. Season with salt and pepper.

3   Turn the heat down to medium, then add the dry mix and cook for a further 4–5 minutes.

4   Now add the wet mix and cook for around 8 minutes or until the vegetables are soft. Add the sesame oil, nam pla and rice wine vinegar and cook for a further 2 minutes.

5   Turn off the heat and allow the mince to cool slightly.

6   Now add the chopped spring onions. You can serve this with lettuce cups or any of my breads on page 162, with a dollop of crème fraîche and lime.

Serves 2

30ml (1fl oz) extra virgin olive oil
400g (14oz) venison mince
200g (7oz) oyster mushrooms, thinly sliced
30g (1oz) salted butter
1 teaspoon sesame oil
1 teaspoon nam pla
1 teaspoon rice wine vinegar
4 spring onions, finely sliced
1 tablespoon crème fraîche
Juice of 1 lime
Flaked sea salt and freshly ground black pepper, to taste

For the dry mix
1 teaspoon ground cumin
1 teaspoon smoked paprika

For the wet mix
2 large shallots, thinly sliced
25g (1oz) minced garlic
20g (¾oz) minced ginger
2 bird's eye chillies, finely sliced

Beef and lettuce burger

Who doesn't love a good burger? This version is made using prime meat from my butcher, and is simply seasoned with salt and pepper. I don't use a bun with this as I prefer to eat fewer carbs, but you can add your favourite toasted bun, if you like. For some reason I am rubbish at eating burgers and sandwiches cleanly, as they always go all over my face, so I always use a knife and fork. I know, I know, very posh....

1   In a mixing bowl, mix the mince with the breadcrumbs and season with salt and pepper to taste. Divide into 4 and roll into balls. Place each ball in between 2 layers of greaseproof paper and use a pan to flatten them into patties. You can either pan fry these on a high heat or cook them on a barbecue or a griddle. Cook for 4 minutes on each side or to your liking.

2   If you like, place each patty on an iceberg leaf and place on each plate, then layer up with the mayonnaise, gherkins, jalapeno and tomatoes, and top with another layer of crispy iceberg lettuce to form the 'bun'.

Serves 2

400g (14oz) best-quality 10%-fat beef mince
20g (½oz) dried fine breadcrumbs
Flaked sea salt and freshly ground black pepper, to taste

To serve (optional)
1 iceberg lettuce, cut down the middle, leaves washed and drained very well
Mayonnaise
Pickled gherkins, sliced
Jalapeño peppers, sliced
Sliced beef tomato seasoned with olive oil, salt and pepper

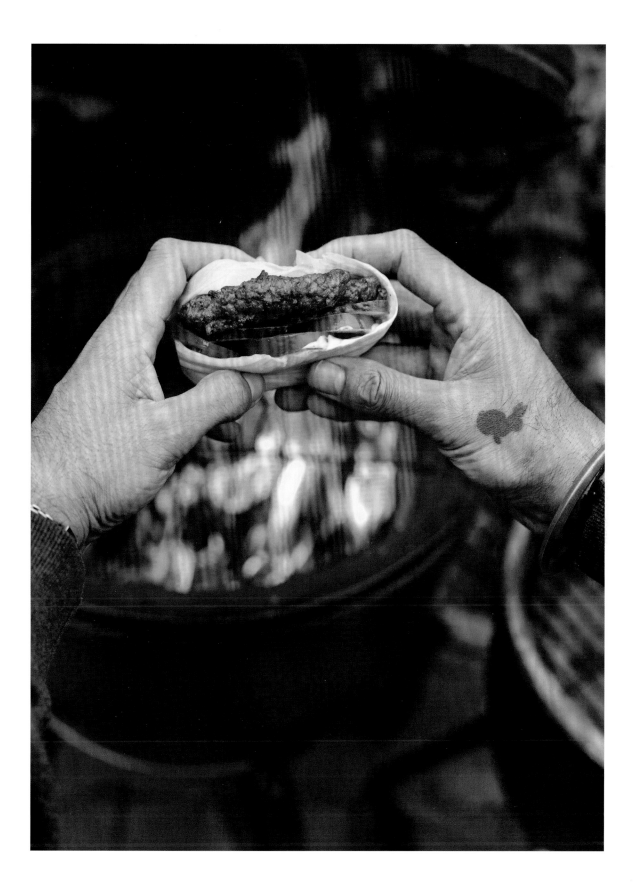

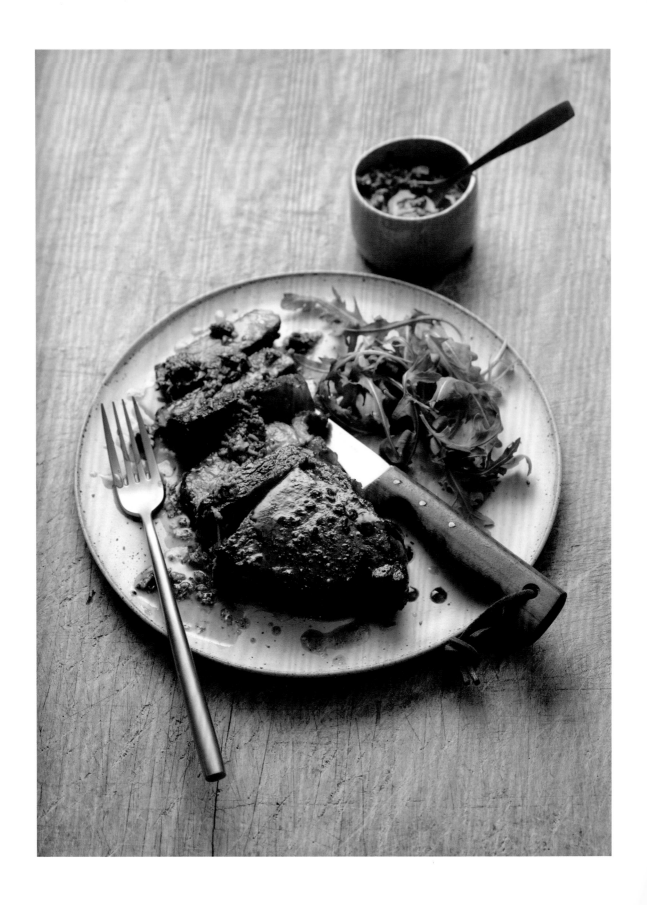

Sirloin steak with my anchovy dressing

The anchovy accompaniment is a brilliant addition to the steak, bringing a salty, fresh, almost salsa-like sauce, while the nuts add a lovely textural contrast.

Equipment | Pestle and mortar

1. Remove the steak from the fridge 30 minutes before cooking.

2. Add all the dressing ingredients, except the lemon juice, oil, capers and parsley, to a pestle and mortar and grind to a smooth paste. Now add the capers, lemon juice and olive oil and fold in the chopped parsley to create a thick, unctuous dressing.

3. Drizzle the steaks with olive oil and season with salt and pepper. Heat a heavy-duty cast-iron pan until smoking hot. Add the steaks and lower the heat to medium–high. Cook the steaks for 1 minute, then turn over. Repeat this for 6–8 minutes to cook the steak to your liking. As a rough guide, the temperature of the steak should be 40°C/104°F for rare, 50°C/122°F for medium rare, 58°C/136°F for medium and 68°C/154°F plus for well done.

4. When cooked, remove from the heat and place on a warm plate, drizzle over the cooking juices from the pan and leave to rest for 10 minutes in a low oven at 90°C/225°F/gas mark ¼ before serving.

5. When ready to serve, pour over the dressing, which should baste and cover the steaks, the heat of the meat releasing all those incredible flavours.

Serves 2

2 x 300g (10oz) sirloin steaks
Extra virgin olive oil, for frying
Flaked sea salt and freshly ground black pepper, to taste

For the dressing
4 anchovy fillets (I use Ortiz)
15g (½oz) pecan nuts, chopped
1 garlic clove
1 teaspoon cayenne pepper
Zest and juice of 1 lemon
½ teaspoon flaked salt
1 teaspoon crushed black pepper
1 teaspoon capers, chopped
50ml (2fl oz) extra virgin olive oil
20g (¾oz) chopped parsley

My four-bean beef chilli

This is a brilliant dish for a cold day when you have time for it to simmer for a couple of hours. You can serve this with lettuce cups with soured cream or, as we do, wholemeal wraps that have been toasted in a dry frying pan, then fill with sliced cucumber, red onion and a small amount of grated mature Cheddar or Gruyère cheese. When you fry the mince, don't be alarmed when bits of the meat stick to the bottom of the pan, just as with my Minced venison and oyster mushroom winter warmer (page 135), the addition of the wet mix will deglaze the pan.

Nutrition notes

Pre-cooked tinned beans in water are extremely healthy, and when packed at source, they retain most of their beneficial nutrients. Diversity is key again, so using four different beans increases their variety and nutrient availability. Beans have long been touted for their heart health, but why is this? Having plenty of beans in our diet can help to reduce cholesterol, manage blood pressure and can help to manage the blood sugar response to eating. Thus they are highly beneficial to managing heart health. Beans are also high in fibre and beneficial plant compounds that the bugs in our guts love and thrive on, which helps to increase the diversity of the gut bacteria, which can have a range of beneficial health effects. We should all be aiming to increase the consumption of a diverse range of beans in our diet.

1   Heat the olive oil in a large saucepan on a medium-high heat, then fry the mince, using a wooden spatula to help break it up while it's cooking. Cook until golden and separated.

2   Add the dry mix and cook for a further 2-3 minutes, then add the wet mix and cook for around 8 minutes or until the meat is tender, scraping up any stuck bits on the bottom of the pan.

3   Add the tomatoes and cook for a further 2 minutes, then pour in the bone broth or chicken stock, bring up to a simmer and add the tin of beans. Reduce the heat to a gentle simmer, cover and cook for 1½-2 hours.

4   Season with salt and pepper to taste and serve topped with the spring onions and with a dollop of soured cream.

Serves 2

30ml (1fl oz) extra virgin olive oil

300g (10oz) lean beef mince

1 x 400g (14oz) tin of chopped plum tomatoes

300ml (10fl oz) Bone broth (page 157) or chicken stock

1 x 400g (14oz) tin of 4-bean mix in water, washed and drained

Flaked sea salt and freshly ground black pepper, to taste

For the dry mix

3 teaspoons ancho chilli flakes

3 teaspoons ground cumin

3 teaspoons smoked paprika

For the wet mix

2 red long peppers, deseeded and cut into 1cm (½in) dice

2 celery sticks, thinly sliced

1 large shallot, thinly sliced

25g (1oz) minced garlic

2 bird's eye chillies, finely sliced

To serve

4 spring onions, finely sliced

1 tablespoon soured cream

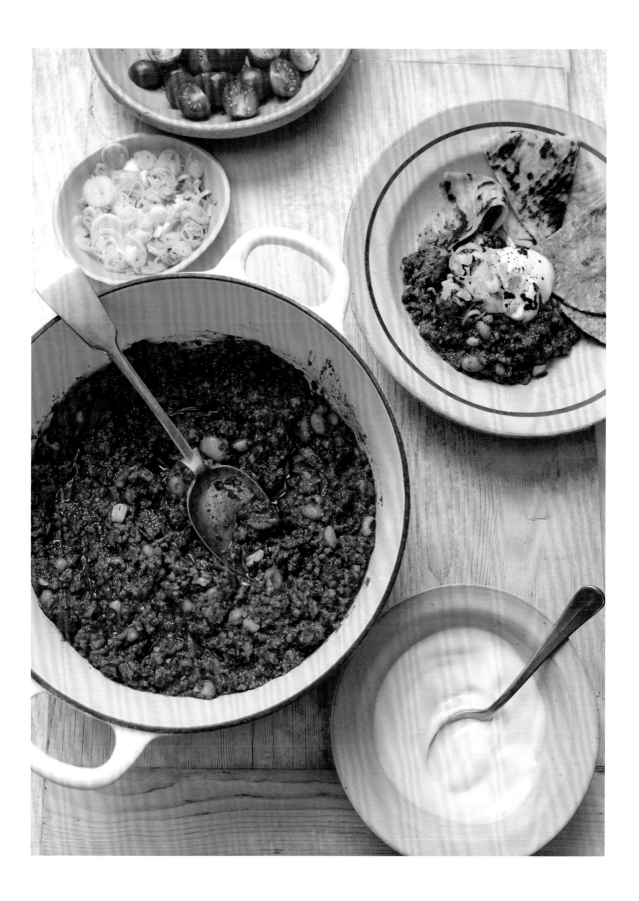

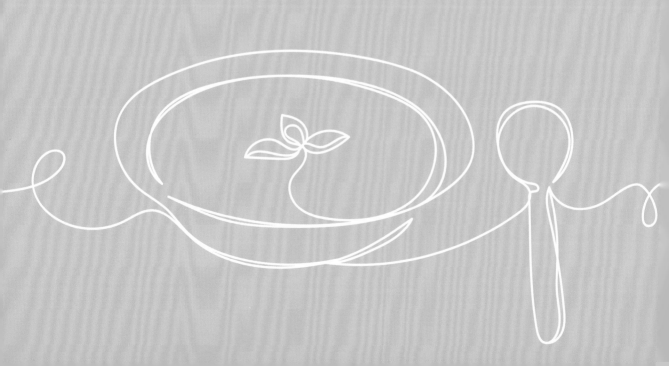

6

soups, sauces, pickles and broths

Cauliflower and almond soup

This soup can be served hot or cold and is delicious with the toasted almonds. It's very clean and the lemon juice adds just a little bit of acidity. Have a jug blender set up, as you will need to purée this soup and pass it through a fine-mesh sieve to create a beautiful velvety texture.

Nutrition notes

Yet again this recipe provides a super tasty opportunity to eat some heart-healthy stars. Cauliflower is a great ingredient to benefit heart health – see page 53. Almonds, too, provide a variety of nutrients to support heart health, including unsaturated fatty acids, vitamin E, phytosterols, copper, magnesium and manganese.

Equipment | Blender

1   Heat the oil in a large heavy-based saucepan. Add the sliced onion and cook gently until tender but with no colour, about 5 minutes. Add the shaved cauliflower and 20g (¾oz) of the almonds and cook for a further 4–5 minutes without colouring. Cover with the water and milk, then simmer for about 15 minutes. Season to taste with salt and pepper and lemon juice.

2   Leave to cool slightly, then blend the soup until very smooth. Pass through a fine-mesh sieve into a clean pan.

3   To serve, reheat gently but don't boil and serve in 2 warm soup bowls. Finely chop the rest of the almonds and sprinkle over the soup, then drizzle with olive oil.

Serves 2

30ml (1fl oz) olive oil, plus extra to serve
1 sweet white onion, very thinly sliced
1 cauliflower, shaved wafer thin
30g (1oz) toasted Marcona almonds
500ml (18fl oz) water
500ml (18fl oz) milk
Juice of 1 lemon, to taste
Flaked sea salt and freshly ground black pepper, to taste

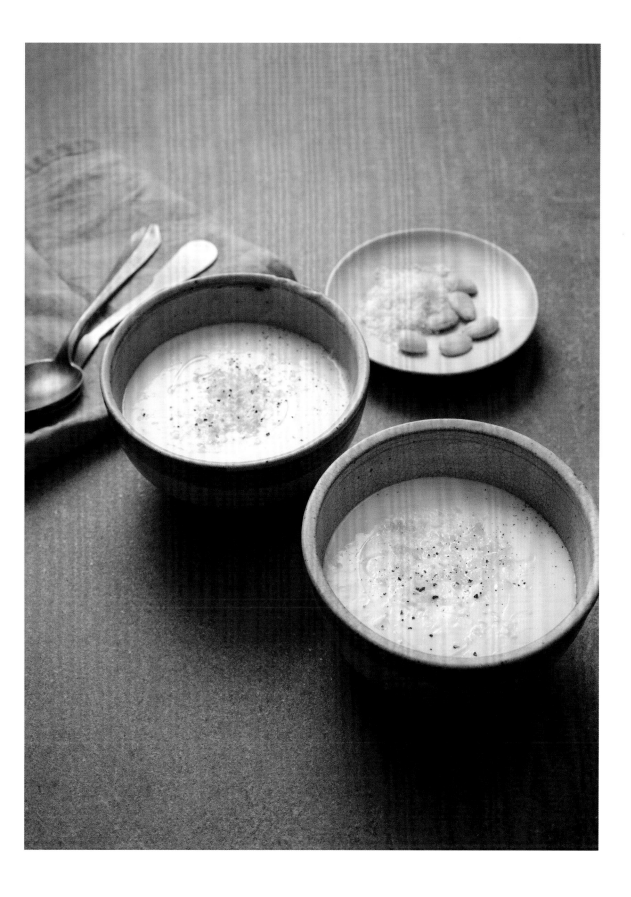

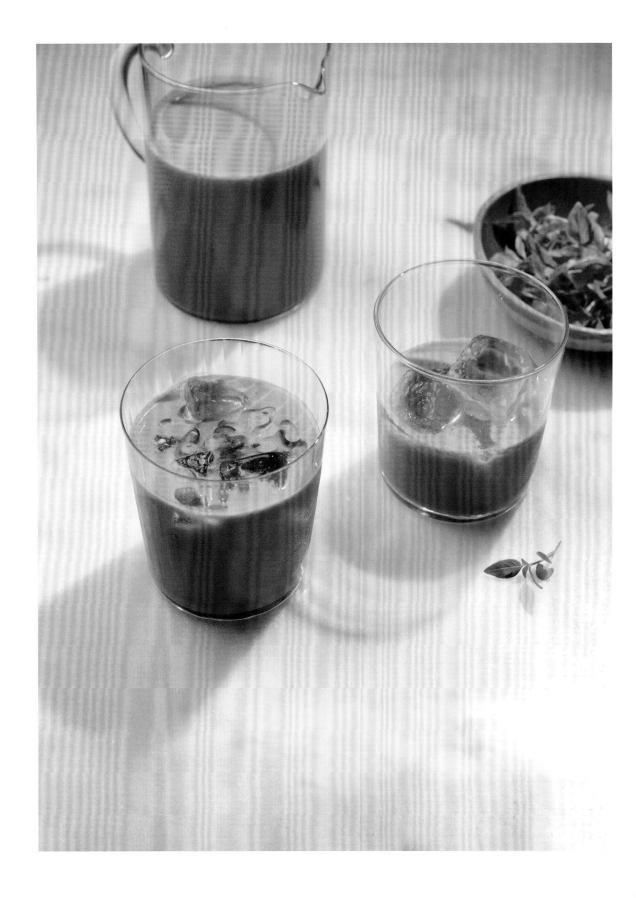

Chilled gazpacho with chilli

This is perfect on a hot summer's day. You can prepare it well in advance and have it ice-cold in the fridge in a flask. Serve it with a couple of ice cubes and a few dried chilli flakes with some hot baked bread drizzled in olive oil for a great temperature contrast.

Nutrition notes

Emerging observational research suggests that eating spicy food regularly could be good for your heart health. For example, a research study found that people who consumed chilli pepper four or more times per week over eight years had significantly lower rates of death, including due to cardiovascular disease. Although this data is intriguing, a cause-and-effect relationship cannot be established yet. That said, the proposed benefits to our health from consuming chillies are thought to be due to capsaicin, the compound that makes them hot. Capsaicin is a potent antioxidant with anti-inflammatory properties.

Equipment | Blender

1   Place all the ingredients except the last 3 into a bowl and mix. Season with the olive oil, sherry vinegar and salt to your liking. Leave for 2 hours to marinate.

2   Place into a blender and blend until smooth, then pass through a fine-mesh sieve. You can add some cold water to lightly loosen the mix, if you like.

3   You can serve this immediately or store it in the fridge in an airtight container, where it will keep for a couple of days. Just remember to blend again before serving, as it can sometimes separate.

Serves 2

400g (14oz) ripe tomatoes, chopped
½ cucumber, peeled and chopped into 5cm (2in) pieces
1 red onion, chopped
2 garlic cloves
1 red pepper, deseeded and chopped
1 small handful of basil
1 bird's eye chilli, deseeded and chopped

45g (1½oz) sourdough bread, crusts removed and torn into pieces
Extra virgin olive oil, to taste
Sherry vinegar, to taste
Flaked sea salt, to taste

Spinach and watercress soup

I first made this over 25 years ago and I still love it; it's smooth and velvety, and the poached egg adds an incredible unctuous element, and the watercress a nice peppery kick. This soup can also be served chilled with the warm poached egg to add the contrast of hot and cold.

Nutrition notes

This recipe combines two great greens: we have spinach from the *Chenopodiaceae* family (also including beetroot and chard) and watercress from the cabbage family, *Brassicaceae*. Both contain high amounts of nitrates. Primarily studied using beetroot juice, dietary nitrate has been shown to support the lowering of blood pressure, which is important for overall cardiovascular health. Watercress is one of the most nutrient-dense edible plants, meaning gram for gram it contains some of the highest quantities of over 50 vital vitamins and minerals. It is exceptionally high in vitamin K, a fat-soluble vitamin necessary for blood clotting and healthy bones, which may reduce the risk of osteoporosis. This is because vitamin K is a component of osteocalcin, a protein that makes up healthy bone tissue and helps regulate bone turnover.

Serves 2

20ml (1fl oz) olive oil
25g (1oz) sliced shallots
500ml (18fl oz) chicken broth or water
50g (2oz) Maris Piper potatoes, thinly sliced
150g (5oz) chopped spinach
150g (5oz) chopped watercress
4 eggs, poached for 3 minutes
Flaked sea salt and freshly ground black pepper, to taste

1 Heat the oil in a large pan, add the sliced shallots and cook for a few minutes until soft but not coloured.

2 Now place the broth or water and the potatoes in the pan with a pinch of salt and bring up to a simmer. Turn the heat down and simmer until the potatoes are cooked, 6–8 minutes. Add the spinach and watercress and cook for a further 2 minutes.

3 Transfer everything to a blender and blend until smooth. Pass through a fine-mesh sieve into a clean pan, bring up to the heat but do not boil, then taste for seasoning.

4 Ladle the soup into 2 warm bowls, top with the poached eggs and enjoy.

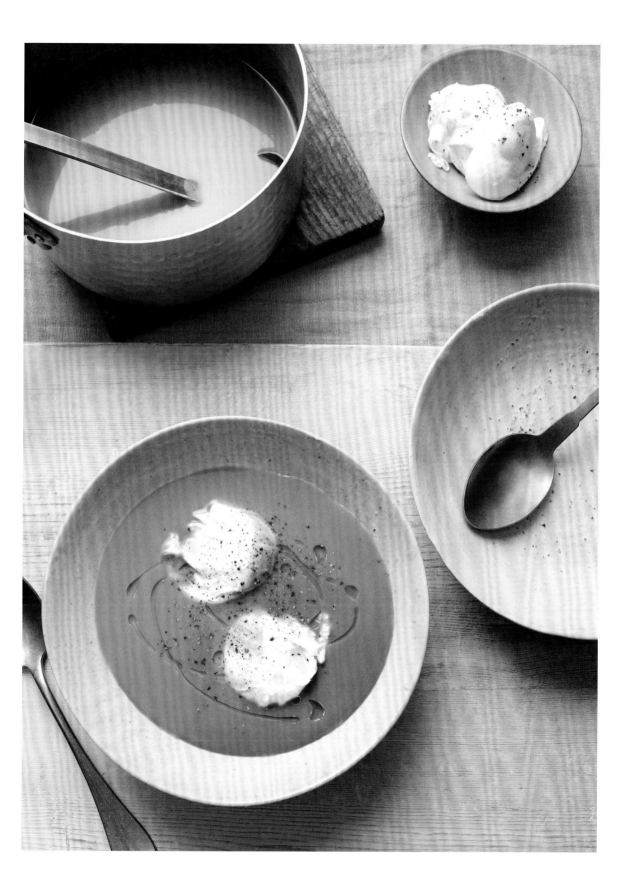

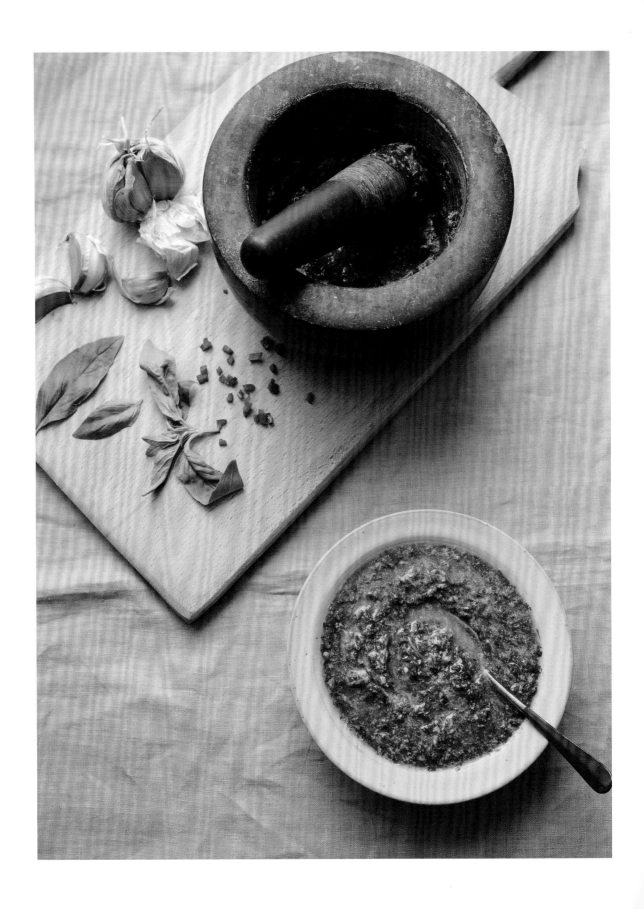

Angus's chimichurri

This recipe is from one of the young chefs in the kitchen: Angus is 20 years old and holds great promise. When I said I would like to use his recipe, he gave me permission - I hope you enjoy it as much as me. On Saturdays I often eat a steak for lunch and Angus makes one of the best chimichurris I have ever tasted: punchy with garlic and Parmesan, it makes the perfect accompaniment smothered all over the hot steak.

Nutrition notes

This recipe provides an excellent opportunity to cram lots of wonderful herbs into a delicious accompaniment. While the purported health benefits of herbs come from studies which either use a mega-dose that is unlikely to be sustainable in a well-balanced diet, or chemical extracts from the plant, consuming fresh herbs will still increase the number of beneficial compounds in your diet. Basil, for example, is a natural source of polyphenols - in particular, phenolic acid (rosmarinic acid) - which can have antioxidant and anti-inflammatory properties.

Interestingly, human perception of coriander's taste can vary dramatically: some describe it as bittersweet or slightly spicy, while others find it soapy with a repugnant odour. Studies now suggest that these individual differences may be due to variations in genes that control our sense of taste and response to the chemical compounds found in foods.

Equipment | Pestle and mortar

1   Place all the herbs and a pinch of salt in a pestle and mortar and crush to a paste. Add the Parmesan, garlic, lime zest and juice and white wine vinegar, and stir to combine. Add the olive oil and red chilli and gently fold through. Season with salt and pepper, if needed.

Serves 2

200g (7oz) basil leaves
150g (5oz) coriander leaves (no stalks, save these for something else)
150g (5oz) flat leaf parsley leaves
70g (3oz) grated Parmesan
½ garlic clove, crushed
Zest and juice of 1 lime

1 teaspoon white wine vinegar
175ml (6fl oz) extra virgin olive oil
1 red chilli, deseeded and finely diced (add the seeds if you like it a bit spicier)
Flaked sea salt and freshly ground black pepper, to taste

Red lentil and lemongrass soup

This lentil soup is an adaptation of the one we serve at the restaurant. It's heavily aromatic with Thai spices and a kick of heat from the chilli. The amount of water in this recipe is deceptive; as a pulse, the lentil can absorb a lot of liquids and once blended, it becomes thicker because the starch is activated, so you will need all that water. Have a jug blender set up, as you will need to purée this soup and pass it through a fine-mesh sieve to create a beautiful velvety texture.

Nutrition notes

Regularly incorporating legumes such as lentils into our diet offers a tasty means to improve our glycaemic control and blood lipids, and to control body weight and reduce metabolic disease risk. Lentils are nutritionally dense, offering a high portion of fibre that slows the rate at which food passes through the gut, making you feel fuller for longer and reducing the glycaemic response to eating. This can support a reduced risk of developing insulin resistance and type 2 diabetes. Despite this, many of us do not consume enough legumes in our diet, so this recipe and others in this book (Roast chicken salad beluga lentils, pickled ginger and sriracha; Momma Bains' chickpea curry; Lentil dhal; Chicken meatballs with butter beans [pages 58, 62, 72, 124]) provide some tasty opportunities to increase our intake and reap the health benefits.

Equipment | Blender

1   Heat the oil and butter in a large heavy-based saucepan on a medium heat until the butter has melted. Add the lentils and sweat for 3-4 minutes until they become translucent. Now add the shallots, ginger, garlic and chillies and cook for another few minutes so they release their flavours.

2   Add the water, bashed lemongrass and the lime leaves and bring to a gentle simmer, this will not take longer than 20 minutes.

3   Once the lentils are cooked, carefully take out the lime leaves and lemongrass and discard. Add some salt and pepper to taste.

4   Now blend the soup in small batches until very smooth; it is important not to overwork otherwise the lentils will become gluey – I would blend for 50–60 seconds each batch. Once blended, pass through a fine-mesh sieve into a clean pan.

5   To serve, reheat the soup but don't let it boil, and garnish with the chopped coriander.

Serves 2

50ml (2fl oz) olive oil
25g (1oz) salted butter
200g (7oz) dried red lentils, washed and drained
2 shallots, finely sliced
15g (½oz) grated ginger
15g (½oz) grated garlic
2 red chillies, finely sliced
2 litres (3½ pints) water
3 lemongrass stalks, bashed to bruise them
5 lime leaves
5g (⅛oz) coriander leaves, chopped, to serve
Flaked sea salt and freshly ground black pepper, to taste

Kimchi

Kimchi is a traditional Korean side dish of salted and fermented vegetables, such as cabbage. A wide selection of seasonings is used, including spring onions, garlic, ginger and chilli. If you buy this, it is important to get hold of raw kimchi, so it doesn't lose the benefits of the fermentation process that gives so much of the gut bacteria goodness.

Nutrition notes

Kimchi has seen an increase in popularity in Western diets due to its reputation for being healthy and providing probiotic bacteria. It is the fermentation process of the vegetables in kimchi that not only alters the flavour, but produces the beneficial probiotic bacteria. There are microbes that naturally occur on the vegetables, and most of the fermentation is due to microbes called lactic acid bacteria. If we eat more fermented food, we can increase the range of good bacteria in the gut, and this has been supported by scientific studies. There is burgeoning research to suggest that regular consumption of certain probiotic bacteria and fermented foods could have a range of health benefits, including regulating the immune system and improving mental health.

Serves 2

1 medium Chinese cabbage (around 1kg/2¼lb), cut into bite-sized pieces
30g (1oz) flaked sea salt
20g (¾oz) sugar
6 garlic cloves, grated
1 thumb-size piece of ginger, grated
4 spring onions, thinly sliced
100g (3½oz) mooli radish, peeled and thinly sliced
20g (¾oz) chilli powder

1   In a large mixing bowl, mix the cabbage and salt together, cover and let the cabbage sit for 2–3 hours, stirring occasionally.

2   In a mixing bowl, combine the sugar, garlic, ginger, spring onions, mooli and chilli powder. Add the cabbage to the chilli paste mixture and use your hands to mix everything together, making sure the cabbage is evenly coated with the paste.

3   Transfer the kimchi to a sterilized Kilner jar, press down on the kimchi to pack it tightly and release any air pockets, then close the lid. Leave the jar at room temperature for 5–7 days to allow the kimchi to ferment. Check every day to release any built-up gas and to taste-test for readiness. Once it reaches your desired level of fermentation, store the jar in the fridge.

Sat's tip: To sterilize, remove the rubber seals and place freshly washed Kilner jars upside down on a deep roasting tray. Place in preheated oven at 160ºC/350ºF for 15 minutes. Wash the rubber seals separately in boiling water for 3 minutes.

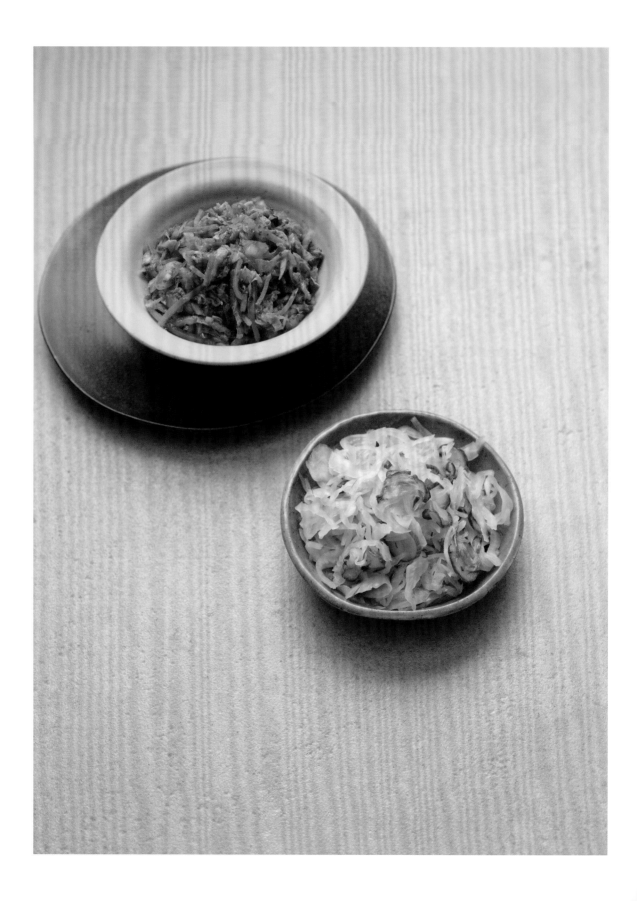

Sauerkraut

Sauerkraut is finely cut raw cabbage that has been fermented by various lactic acid bacteria. It has a long shelf life and a distinctive sour flavour, both of which result from the lactic acid formed when the bacteria ferment the sugars in the cabbage leaves. It is one of the best-known national dishes in Germany and Eastern Europe. I have it with lots of things, from pork chops to steaks.

Nutrition notes

This recipe provides the opportunity to make your own sauerkraut to get the proposed health benefits of fermented foods. This recipe is important, as often shop-bought canned sauerkraut undergoes sterilizations so it no longer contains live bacteria. Fermented foods have been around for thousands of years, and there is growing evidence for their health benefits. Scientists define fermented foods as those made through desired microbial growth and enzymatic conversions of food components. Many of the species of bacteria that are produced in fermented foods such as sauerkraut are similar to probiotic bacteria, such as Lactobacillus plantarum, which can support gut health, reducing the risk of gastrointestinal infections and improving immunity.

Serves 2

1 medium white cabbage
(roughly 1kg/2¼lb),
finely sliced
25g (1oz) flaked sea salt

1   In a large mixing bowl, combine the sliced cabbage and sea salt. Using your hands, massage the cabbage for 5–10 minutes until it starts to release its liquid; this will help create the brine in which the sauerkraut will ferment.

2   Pack the cabbage tightly into a sterilized Kilner jar (see Sat's tip on page 153), pressing down firmly with your fists as you go to release any air bubbles. Pour any remaining liquid from the mixing bowl into the jar, making sure the cabbage is fully submerged. Place the lid on the jar and store it in a cool dark place.

3   Check the sauerkraut every few days to make sure the cabbage is still submerged under the brine. After 1 week, taste the sauerkraut to see if it is sour enough – this comes down to personal taste – if you like it more sour, leave for a couple more days until it's ready.

4   When the sauerkraut is ready, place in the fridge. It will last for several months.

Dashi

I first came across dashi on my first trip to Japan in 2007, and it blew me away – full of umami (see page 12), amino acids and mouth-filling deliciousness. It is very healthy and clean, and it makes a nourishing drink; or add some noodles and a couple of poached eggs and you have a more substantial meal. You can also freeze this and use it as a base for soups.

Umami is the fifth taste, basically something us humans have a predisposition to. It's a natural MSG that's found in specific foods like tomatoes, anchovies, Parmesan, meat and fish and is also found in abundance in mothers' milk, so we get a taste for it from a very early age. Translated it means deliciousness, and is packed full of amino acids and MSG. I use dashi a lot in cooking at the restaurant and at home, which also means I can reduce the extra salt in certain dishes too.

Nutrition notes

The Japanese people are known for their longevity, and their unique diet is believed to contribute to this good health. That said, there is no magic bullet here, and the health properties of Japanese cuisine is likely multifaceted due to the diversity of fish, fruits, vegetables, seaweed, soya bean foods, fermented foods and the soup stock 'dashi' that forms the diet. Dashi is a principal component, and the combination of kombu seaweed (which is high in iodine, potassium, calcium, iron, potassium, magnesium, zinc and vitamins B, C, D and E) and bonito flakes (high in essential amino acids) could be contributing factors to the health benefits of its regular consumption. Indeed, daily consumption of dried bonito flake broth was shown to lower blood pressure in healthy elderly participants.

Equipment | Food thermometer probe

2 litres (3½ pints) mineral water
50g (2oz) kombu seaweed
20g (¾oz) bonito flakes
75ml (3fl oz) soy sauce
30ml (1fl oz) mirin
25ml (1fl oz) rice wine vinegar

1 Heat the water and kombu in a large pan over a medium heat up to around 75°C/170°F. Pull the pan off the heat and add the bonito flakes, then allow to stand for 3 minutes. Pass the liquid through a fine-mesh sieve and add the soy, mirin and rice wine vinegar.

2 Store in the fridge in an airtight container until needed.

Bone broth

This a great source of nourishment for me, I have this during the day and it is surprisingly filling. The secret is to blend it before drinking so the chicken fat emulsifies with the liquor. I sometimes add a few drops of Tabasco at the end to give it a pep.

Equipment | Pressure cooker

1   Wash the vegetables, then place all the ingredients except the soy sauce into the pressure cooker. Cover with the water. Put the lid on and bring up to full pressure. Cook for 2 hours, after which time allow the pressure cooker to cool down naturally and don't open the valve yet.

2   When the liquid is cool enough to remove the lid, remove and strain through a fine-mesh sieve. Store in the fridge or freezer until needed.

3   When serving, allow 250-300ml (8-10fl oz) per person, bring the liquid to a simmer and serve, adding a spoon of soy sauce to each cup.

1 carrot, roughly chopped
½ leek, sliced
1 bulb of garlic, split
    lengthways
2 celery sticks, roughly
    chopped
1 white onion, finely sliced
1 small bunch of thyme
2kg (4½lb) cornfed chicken
    wings, chopped in half
    (ask your butcher to do
    this for you)
3 litres (5 pints) water
50ml (2fl oz) soy sauce,
    to serve

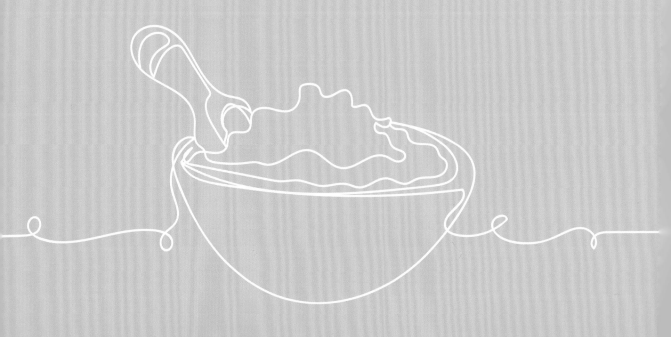

7

smoothies, snacks and breads

My high-protein smoothie

This is perfect after a workout or if you are in a rush and can't stop for brekky. I make this the night before and keep it in a flask in the fridge ready to grab and go. I make the almond milk myself in advance to save time, and also because then I know it won't have any additives in; it is very healthy as a milk substitute with its high protein level. You can make the milk in batches and store it in the fridge for when it is needed.

Equipment | Blender

1 Soak the almonds overnight in a bowl of water. Drain.

2 Place the drained almonds in a blender with the ice-cold water and blend for 2–3 minutes. Strain through a fine-mesh sieve and set aside in the fridge, preferably overnight.

3 Place the almond milk, peanut butter, honey and banana in a blender and blend on full power for 30 seconds. Add the ice and blend again for 30 seconds.

4 Pour into chilled glasses and serve.

Serves 2

For the almond milk
75g (3oz) almonds, skin on
325ml (11fl oz) ice-cold water

For the smoothie
30g (1oz) peanut butter
15g (½oz) wild raw honey
1 medium banana
100g (3½oz) ice cubes

Spinach and almond smoothie

This does sound like a lot of spinach but, as it is over 90 per cent water and raw, it provides all the nutrients you need. I have this mid-morning as a snack and it fills me up until my next meal.

🫁 **Nutrition notes**

Spinach is an extremely nutrient-rich vegetable, packed full of compounds called nitrates that play an important role in our heart health. Nitrates help improve blood flow and blood pressure by relaxing the blood vessels, reducing the stiffness of our arteries and promoting dilation. A reduction in blood pressure helps reduce the risk of heart disease and stroke. Recent observational evidence indicates that if we have a higher long-term dietary intake of nitrate, we can lower our risk of cardiovascular disease. Almonds are also rich in nutrients that help protect the heart, including unsaturated fatty acids, vitamin E, phytosterols, copper, magnesium and manganese. Research studies have shown that including almonds in our diet may reduce the risk of heart disease, specifically in overweight individuals. Further research shows that almond consumption helps to reduce LDL cholesterol (bad cholesterol), so this too can help to reduce the risk of heart disease.

Equipment | Blender

1 Place all the ingredients except the ice in a blender and blend on full power for 30 seconds. Add the ice and blend again for 30 seconds.

2 Pour into chilled glasses and serve.

Serves 2

400ml (14fl oz) homemade almond milk (see opposite)
200g (7oz) raw spinach
50g (2oz) wild raw honey
100g (3½oz) ice cubes

Potato flatbread

This recipe is the one I use to accompany my Flattened lamb kofta/kebab (page 130), it is great with my Hummus (page 165) too and versatile enough to have instead of chapattis with any of Momma Bains' curries.

Serves 2

250g (9oz) Maris Piper potatoes
25g (1oz) salted butter
25g (1oz) plain flour
Flaked sea salt, to taste

1   Preheat the oven to 200°C/425°F/gas mark 7.

2   Place the potatoes on a roasting tray and cook in the oven until tender, for around 10–15 minutes.

3   Remove from the oven, cool a little and cut in half. Scoop out the potatoes into a bowl, discarding the skin. Weigh out 200g (7oz) of the potato flesh. Season with a little salt and add the butter and flour. Mix well, cover and leave to rest for 1 hour.

4   Take 50g (2oz) of the mix, place between 2 sheets of greaseproof paper, then roll it out to a depth of around 4mm (0.2in) and repeat until you've used all the mixture. Cook the flatbreads in a hot pan in the greaseproof paper until golden brown on both sides, removing the paper once cooked.

Wholemeal flatbread

The trouble with supermarket-bought wraps is they have lots of ingredients to give them an unnatural shelf life, which can't be good for you. This is a healthy, easy and quick recipe, and these flatbreads will keep in the freezer once cooked, so make in batches and defrost as needed.

Serves 2

120g (4oz) wholemeal flour
½ teaspoon salt
½ teaspoon baking powder
1 tablespoon olive oil
90ml (3fl oz) warm water

1   In a mixing bowl, combine the wholemeal flour, salt and baking powder, and mix well. Then add the olive oil and warm water to the mixing bowl and stir until the dough comes together.

2   Turn the dough out onto a floured surface and knead for 2–3 minutes, until it becomes smooth and elastic, then divide into 4 equal pieces.

3   Using a rolling pin, roll each piece of dough into a circle, about 15–18cm (6-7 inches) in diameter.

4   Heat a non-stick pan over medium-high heat and cook the flatbread in the pan for 1 minute on each side, until it becomes lightly browned and puffed up.

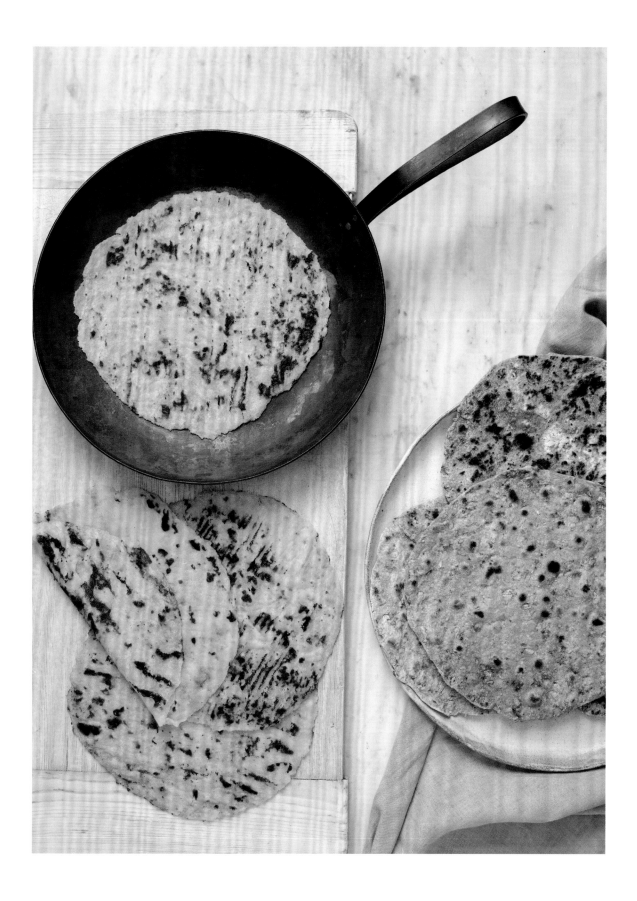

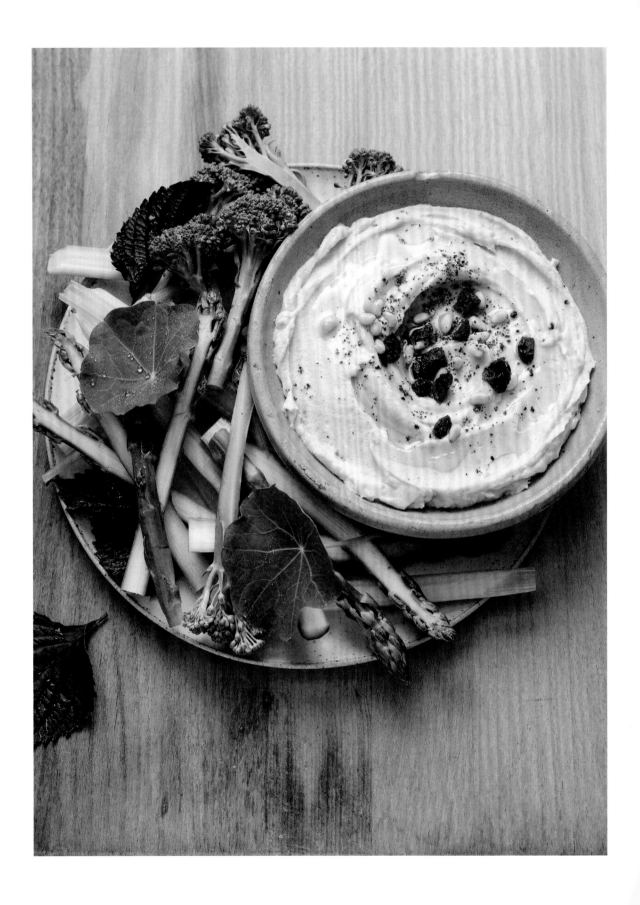

Hummus

Hummus is one of my favourite dips; I love it on roast potatoes, with warm Potato flatbread (page 162) and especially with Crudités (page 40). I always have some in the fridge but if not, I sometimes use the Leon brand, as it is also delicious.

Nutrition notes

Hummus provides a nutritious fibre source and plant-based protein thanks to the powerful chickpea. Chickpeas are especially high in a soluble fibre called raffinose, which can positively alter the type of bugs living in our guts to help promote intestinal health. Furthermore, in general, increased consumption of soluble fibre from foods results in reduced-serum total cholesterol and bad LDL cholesterol (LDL-C) and has an inverse correlation with coronary heart disease mortality. So increasing our intake of pulses such as chickpeas in our diet will be great for our heart health.

Equipment | Blender

1 Place all the ingredients except the pine nuts, sumac, dried cranberries and seasoning in a blender, then blend on full until puréed. Season with a little salt and pepper, if needed. Spoon into a bowl and set aside.

2 Place the pine nuts in a frying pan set over a medium heat. Gently toast for a few minutes until they are golden brown all over. Remove from the heat and sprinkle the sumac over the nuts.

3 Scatter the pine nuts and dried cranberries over the hummus and drizzle over a little olive oil to finish.

Serves 2

250g (9oz) tinned chickpeas (drained weight)
50ml (2fl oz) water
1 small garlic clove
60g (2oz) tahini
30ml (1fl oz) extra virgin olive oil, plus a little extra to drizzle
30ml (1fl oz) lemon juice
¼ teaspoon smoked paprika
40g (1½oz) pine nuts
¼ teaspoon ground sumac
20g (¾oz) dried cranberries
Flaked sea salt and freshly ground black pepper, to taste

Red pepper and onion frittata with tomato salsa

The raw tomato salsa is brilliant as it's quick to make and has a massive punch. I sometimes have the salsa on toast with a fried egg and smashed avocado, or serve it alongside my Flattened lamb kofta/kebab (page 130). The secret of this dish is slow and low cooking and keeping the eggs nice and soft.

⚭ **Nutrition notes**

Red peppers are high in carotenoids – compounds that give vegetables their red and orange colours. The carotenoids lutein and zeaxanthin, when eaten in adequate amounts, support eye health (in much the same way as carrots are reputed to do!). Red peppers are high in capsanthin, a polyphenol that some research suggests can, in significant quantities, support gut health. They also provide an excellent source of potassium, vitamin C and folate, more so than their yellow and green counterparts, although it's worth noting that green peppers contain the highest amounts of polyphenols. Red onion provides another source of colour compounds to our diet. It is also high in non-digestible carbohydrates known as oligosaccharides, which can help feed and support the good bacteria in our guts and so help improve our overall health.

Serves 2

For the tomato salsa
2 ripe plum tomatoes
50g (2oz) red onion, finely
    diced
Pinch of dried chilli flakes
Extra virgin olive oil, to
    drizzle
20g (¾oz) fresh coriander

For the frittata
50ml (2fl oz) olive oil
100g (3½oz) red onion,
    thinly sliced
100g (3½oz) red pepper,
    deseeded and thinly
    sliced
6 large organic eggs
Flaked sea salt and freshly
    ground black pepper, to
    taste

1   First make the salsa. Cut the tomatoes into quarters, then quarters again. Place in a bowl along with the diced red onion. Season with the chilli, olive oil and a pinch of salt. Leave to marinate for 1 hour at room temperature.

2   Heat the oil in a non-stick frying pan over a medium heat and cook the onion and pepper until soft and very tender, 10-15 minutes.

3   Crack the eggs into a bowl and whisk. Add the eggs to the pan and slowly stir until they start to set, then bring the outside of the mixture into the middle of the pan using a spatula. When the mix starts to firm up, turn the heat down and let the mix set.

4   Remove from the heat and slide the frittata on to a warm plate.

5   Chop the coriander and mix it into the tomatoes, then spoon over the frittata and serve.

Eat To Your Heart's Content

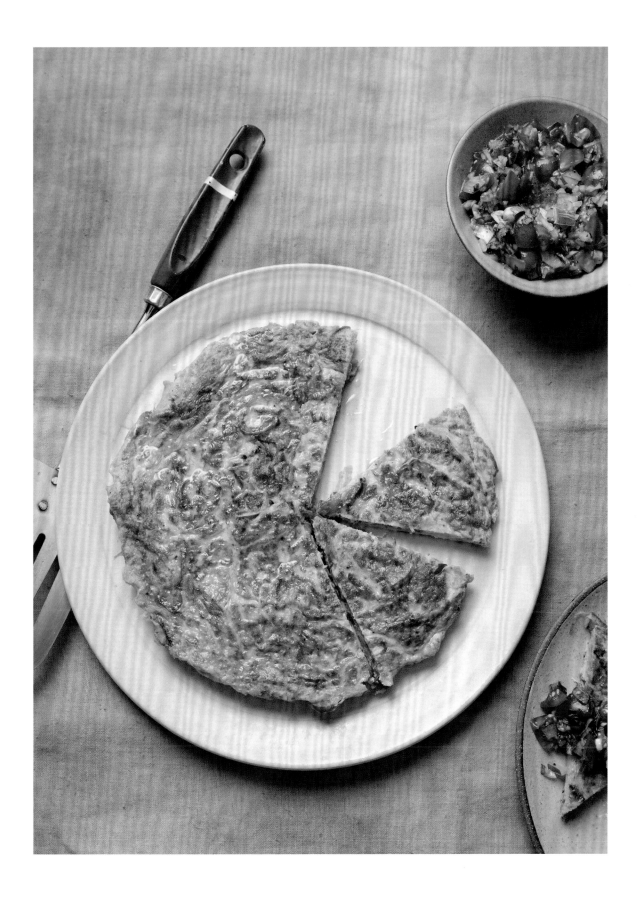

Olive oil shot

Me and my head chef John have this each morning before we eat, as it is a great source of antioxidants and mono-unsaturated fatty acids, which have been associated with a reduced risk of heart disease.

Nutrition notes

Olive oil is the main source of fat within the Mediterranean diet, a diet that has been linked with Blue Zones (pockets of the world where populations have the longest life expectancy). Although a Mediterranean diet is very diverse, a contributing factor to the health benefits could be the high intake of olive oil. Olive oil is rich in antioxidants and mono-unsaturated fatty acids. Most people will get plenty of these benefits from using olive oil in cooking, however, if you don't routinely cook with it, then a shot may be an alternative option. A review of the available evidence suggested that there may be an overall risk reduction in cardiovascular disease when comparing a high intake of mono-unsaturated fatty acids to a lower one.

1   Place all the ingredients in a jug and stir to combine.

2   Pour into shot glasses and drink in one.

Serves 2

4 tablespoons olive oil
Juice of 1 lemon
½ teaspoon cayenne pepper
60g (2oz) honey

168   Eat To Your Heart's Content

Braised nuts

This is a great alternative to grains or pulses, and it goes really well with any dishes that accompany pasta or rice, such as the Venison chilli with bitter chocolate (page 134). Using the pressure cooker gives a lovely texture to these nuts, allowing them to swell and almost become creamy when full of the stock and flavours.

Nutrition notes

Nuts should form a routine staple for our diverse heart-healthy diet; they are an excellent source of unsaturated fats and contain an excellent amount of fibre that can help reduce cholesterol being absorbed into the bloodstream from the gut. They are also relatively high in protein, vitamin E, magnesium and potassium. This nutrient makeup is why epidemiologic studies have associated nut consumption with a reduced incidence of coronary heart disease. One study of note showed that a Mediterranean diet supplemented with 30g (1oz) of mixed nuts (walnuts, almonds and hazelnuts) per day resulted in beneficial effects on blood lipid profile in diabetic and non-diabetic participants. We could all aim to increase our intake to 30g (1oz) per day from a variety of types, so this recipe helps to provide that opportunity.

Equipment | Pressure cooker

1 Warm both chicken stocks and the soy sauce in a pressure cooker. Add the nuts and put the lid on. Bring up to full pressure and cook for 10 minutes.

2 Turn off the pressure and allow the pan to cool naturally, without opening the vent. Remove the lid and season with a little salt if necessary.

Serves 2

100g (3½oz) white chicken stock
100g (3½oz) brown chicken stock
20g (¾oz) soy sauce
50g (2oz) pine nuts
50g (2oz) pistachios
50g (2oz) hazelnuts
Flaked sea salt, to taste

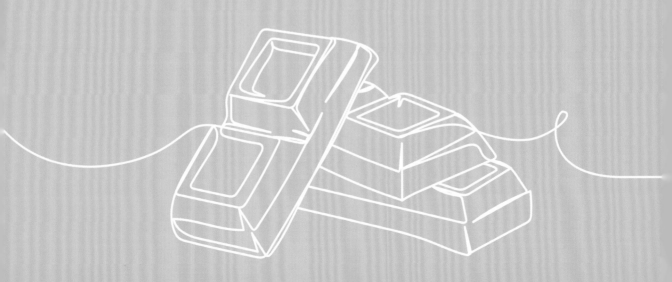

8

sweet
things

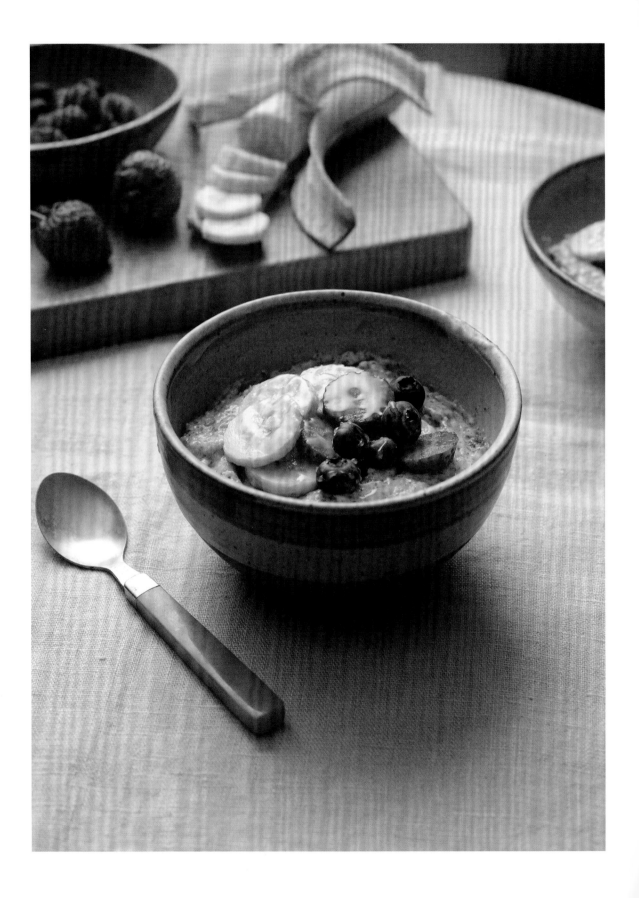

Porridge with nuts, seeds and fruit

I grew up eating porridge and have always loved it, but adding seeds, nuts and fruit gives it a lovely texture. Add your favourite nuts and seeds to make it more bespoke to you.

1 Place all the porridge ingredients in a pan over a medium–high heat. Bring to a simmer, turn the heat down to medium and start whisking. Whisk for 2 minutes, and by this time the porridge should have started to thicken up. Remove from the heat and rest for 2 minutes. If the porridge is a little thick, just add a splash of milk.

2 Place the strawberries, raspberries and blueberries in a pan and gently warm over a medium heat until the berries just start to bleed. Remove from the heat and add the banana slices, then set aside until needed.

3 Distribute the porridge evenly between 2 bowls and spoon over the berries and banana. If you like it a touch sweeter, drizzle with a little more Manuka honey.

Serves 2

50g (2oz) jumbo porridge oats
20g (¾oz) Manuka honey, plus extra to serve (optional)
500ml (18fl oz) milk
25g (1oz) sunflower seeds
50g (2oz) mixed nuts, skin on
25g (1oz) flaxseeds
25g (1oz) sultanas

For the berries
50g (2oz) strawberries, quartered
50g (2oz) raspberries
50g (2oz) blueberries
1 medium banana, sliced

RSB overnight oats with seeds and nuts

This recipe is the same one that we use at RSB for our guests that have stayed over with us, and it is very popular. You will notice that we don't use a lot of honey, and that is because the fruits used add a natural sweetness to the dish.

⚛ Nutrition notes

As mentioned in Porridge with nuts, seeds and fruits (page 173), porridge oats contain beta-glucan, which is a soluble fibre that is found in the outer cell wall of oats. The beta-glucan in porridge oats can support our appetite control in two ways. One, as beta-glucan partially dissolves it forms a thick, gel-like solution in your gut, delaying the time it takes for your stomach to empty; two, beta-glucan increases the release of peptide YY, a satiety hormone, which can lead to reduced calorie intake and may decrease our risk of obesity.

There is more, too, with beta-glucan increasing the growth of good bacteria in the gut, which have a wide range of positive health benefits.

1 Mix all the ingredients together in a bowl. Place into a container and store in the fridge overnight.

Serves 2

75g (3oz) porridge oats
50g (2oz) natural yoghurt
125ml (4fl oz) apple juice
½ teaspoon ground
    cinnamon
100g (3½oz) raisins
1 Granny Smith apple,
    grated with the skin on
1 tablespoon flaxseeds
1 tablespoon sunflower
    seeds

1 tablespoon flaked
    almonds
10ml (¼fl oz) wild raw
    honey

Greek yoghurt with strawberries, mint and olive oil

This hits the spot for me when I'm craving something sweet, and it allows me to keep an eye on my sweet tooth. If you fancy something a little more decadent, try adding some grated 70+ per cent cocoa solids chocolate over the dish before you eat. The olive oil may sound strange but, trust me, it adds a lovely fruitiness and creaminess.

Nutrition notes

Heart disease is the most common cause of death worldwide. Studies have found a relationship between the regular consumption of berries rich in anthocyanins and improved heart health. It is these anthocyanins that give strawberries their rich red colour. Strawberries may also reduce inflammation, improve vascular function, improve blood lipids and reduce harmful oxidation of bad (LDL) cholesterol. A vibrant, heart-healthy food.

1 Divide the yoghurt between 2 bowls.

2 Mix together the strawberries, mint and basil, and sweeten it up with the honey. Spoon on top of the yoghurt and drizzle over a little olive oil.

Serves 2

300g (10oz) thick Greek
   yoghurt
200g (7oz) strawberries,
   cut in half
5g (⅛oz) mint leaves, torn
5g (⅛oz) basil leaves, torn
30ml (1fl oz) wild raw
   honey
20ml (¾fl oz) extra virgin
   olive oil

Chocolate protein cookies

We all need something sweet in our life, and I am no exception, so if we are going eat something sweet, let's make it delicious and healthy too. These are my protein cookies; they last up to a week in the fridge and I use either Huel or PhD as a protein source.

Equipment | 2 x 30cm x 22cm x 2.5cm (12in x 9in x 1in) baking trays

1   Preheat the oven to 180°C/400°F/gas mark 6. Line the baking trays with greaseproof paper.

2   Place all the ingredients except the chocolate drops into a mixing bowl. Mix to a dough, then add in the chocolate drops. Divide the mixture into 12 balls and place on the baking trays. Bake for 12 minutes.

3   Remove from the oven and use the back of a fork to gently press the cookies down. Transfer to a wire rack and leave to cool. Store in an airtight container until ready to eat.

Makes 12 cookies

250g (9oz) chunky peanut butter
75g (3oz) honey
1 large egg
75g (3oz) chocolate whey protein powder
100ml (3½fl oz) milk
40g (1½oz) white chocolate drops

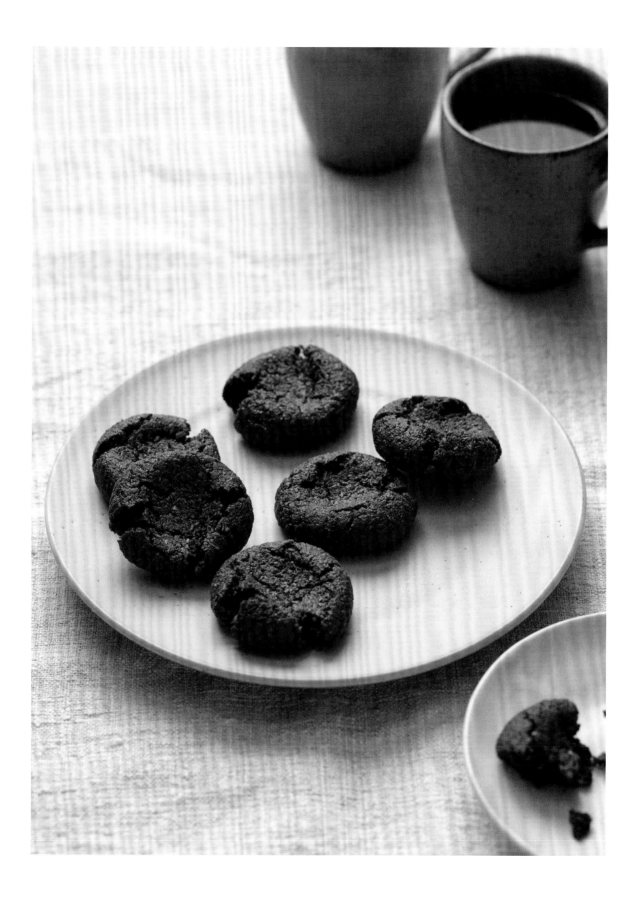

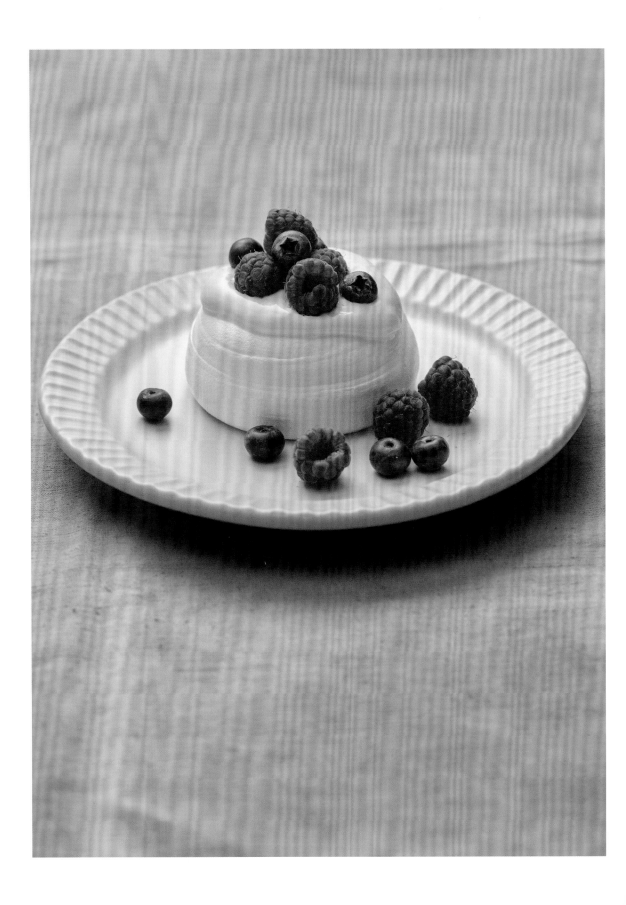

Meringues with raspberries, blueberries and crème fraîche

Meringues are a great way to have something sweet, and using natural honey and raw cane sugar rather than processed sugar is a better way to get a sweet hit. I like to smash my meringues all over the crème fraîche and berries so I get lovely crispy bits in each spoonful.

Serves 2

50g (2oz) blueberries
50g (2oz) raspberries
125g (4½oz) crème fraîche

For the meringues
35ml (1oz) water
85g (3oz) honey
85g (3oz) raw cane sugar
110g (4oz) egg whites

1 Place the blueberries in a pan and gently warm until they just start to burst. Remove from the heat and fold in the raspberries. Transfer to a bowl, cover and place in the fridge until needed.

2 Preheat the oven to 90°C/225°F/gas mark ¼.

3 Bring the water, honey and sugar to the boil in a pan over a high heat for 5 minutes.

4 In a clean bowl, whisk the egg whites using an electric whisk, while slowly adding the honey syrup, until they are frothy. When fully combined, whisk until the mix cools down a little, about 3 minutes.

5 When cool, place dollops of meringue onto a baking sheet lined with greaseproof paper – you can do these to whatever shape and size you like. Place in the oven for 6 hours or overnight, then check to make sure they are dry (this will depend on what size you have done). If they need a little longer, check every 15 minutes.

6 You can either crush the meringue or serve them whole; it's up to you. Top a meringue nest with some crème fraîche, spoon over the fruit and serve.

Affogato with vanilla ice cream and olive oil

I know, I know, this sounds crazy, but trust me, if I am at a restaurant and really fancy a dessert but not a massive piece of cake or pudding, I always ask for an espresso and a ball of very good-quality ice cream, as this fulfils my sweet craving. The drizzle of olive oil here gives it an incredibly creamy mouthfeel. I will, and do, use shop-bought ice cream for this, just make sure it is of the highest quality.

Nutrition notes

Regular consumption of coffee can increase your intake of antioxidants, which help prevent and repair damage to cells and genetic material around your body. Coffee is a significant source of polyphenols – a type of antioxidant which can help look after the beneficial bacteria in the gut.

1   This can't be any easier: pour 2 cups of espresso into warm coffee cups, add a ball of soft ice cream and drizzle with olive oil.

Serves 2

2 cups of espresso
2 scoops of vanilla ice
    cream
A drizzle of extra virgin
    olive oil

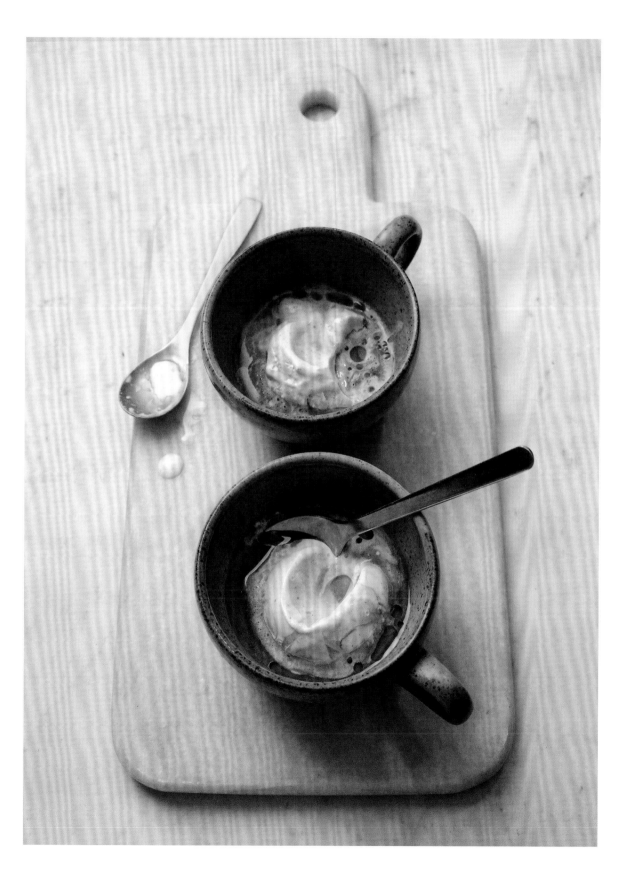

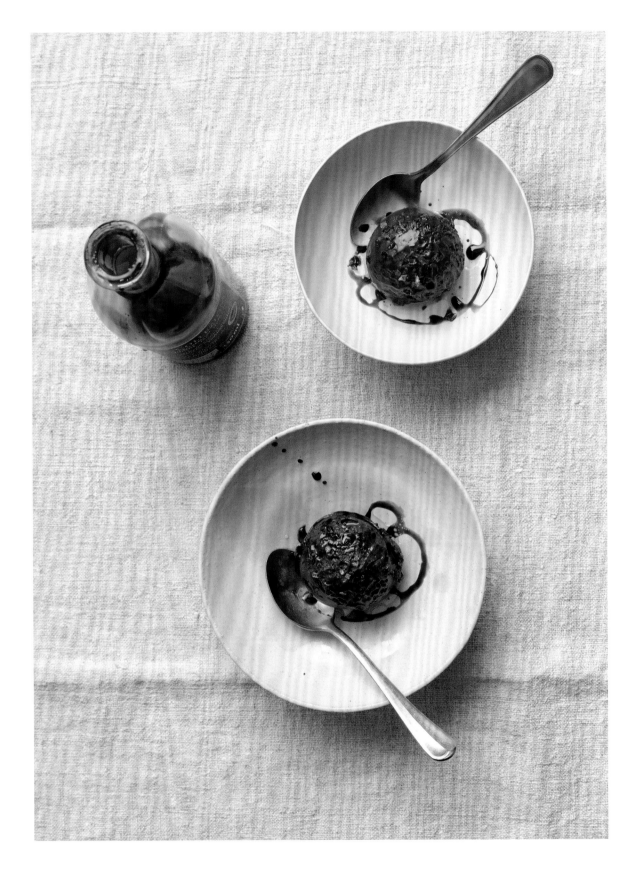

Chocolate mousse with aged balsamic vinegar

My chocolate craving started when I was a young boy. When I worked at my dad's shop I would nick bars of chocolate as a reward, as he never paid me. My fave was Dairy Milk. Now I know that's not the most gourmet bar, but this mousse gives me a chocolate hit to stop me craving the cheaper stuff, which, by the way, I still crave and I am allowed 2 Freddo bars a week on Neil's advice – ha ha! A very simple bitter chocolate recipe, this gives me my cocoa hit and adding the salt, vinegar and olive oil almost brings out so many complexities in the chocolate. Make sure you use super-fresh eggs for this dish.

Nutrition notes

The news we all want to hear... chocolate can be good for us! High-cocoa-content chocolate is rich in antioxidants, which are compounds in some foods that can help prevent damage to the cells in our body. The types found in cocoa are called polyphenols and although some polyphenols are lost during the production process, some cocoa powders still have more antioxidants than so-called superfruits. A specific group of polyphenols in chocolate with heart-health properties are flavanols. Research has linked flavanols to improved blood vessel function and reduced blood pressure, which are important for heart health. Lastly, cocoa is also a prebiotic, a type of fibre that your gut bacteria digest, which increases the growth and activity of beneficial good gut bacteria that can confer a health benefit.

1   Melt the chocolate in the microwave in short bursts, say 10 seconds at a time, until melted.

2   In a clean bowl, whip the egg whites to soft peaks. In another bowl, whisk the egg yolks into the melted and slightly cooled chocolate.

3   Fold in the egg whites and transfer to the fridge to set for at least 3 hours.

4   To serve, remove from the fridge and scoop out a nice portion into a bowl and drizzle with the olive oil and a pinch of salt.

5   When serving, drizzle over the olive oil and some aged balsamic vinegar and sprinkle a little sea salt on top.

Serves 2

200g (7oz) dark chocolate
    (70% cocoa solids)
6 egg whites
2 egg yolks

To serve
Good-quality aged
    balsamic vinegar (I use
    a 25-year-old)
Extra virgin olive oil
Sea salt flakes (I use
    Maldon)

Protein bar

We devised this bar at the restaurant as a little snack to give the team a boost during service. It's great if you're in a rush and you need a little energy boost. I have this post training, so I always have some at home and at work for emergencies.

◌ **Nutrition notes**

Proteins form the essential building blocks of life. Protein helps repair and build our body's tissues, allows metabolic reactions to take place and coordinates bodily functions. Proteins are important for maintaining proper pH and fluid balance. Finally, they keep our immune system strong and transport and store nutrients. Collectively, these functions make protein an essential nutrient for our health.

Equipment | 2 x 20cm x 15cm x 2.5cm (8in x 6in x 1in) baking trays

1   Line one of your baking trays with greaseproof paper.

2   Place the peanut butter, maple syrup and milk in a large, heavy-based pan. Bring to a gentle simmer.

3   Remove from the heat and whisk in the porridge oats, cocoa powder, protein powder, nuts and dried fruit. Add the chocolate drops and press the mixture into the baking tray.

4   Place a sheet of greaseproof on top, followed by another baking tray (this is not essential but it helps to even out the mixture while it's chilling). Place a weight on top – such as a few tins – and chill in the fridge for 2 hours until set. Cut into 16 equal bars before serving.

Makes 12 bars

125g (4½oz) peanut butter
150g (5½oz) maple syrup
25ml (1fl oz) milk
150g (5½oz) ground
    porridge oats
25g (1oz) bitter cocoa
    powder
35g (1¼oz) vanilla protein
    powder
40g (1½oz) shelled
    pistachios
40g (1½oz) flaked
    almonds

60g (2¼oz) dried sultanas
60g (2¼oz) dried cherries
125g (4½oz) chocolate
    drops (70% cocoa
    solids)

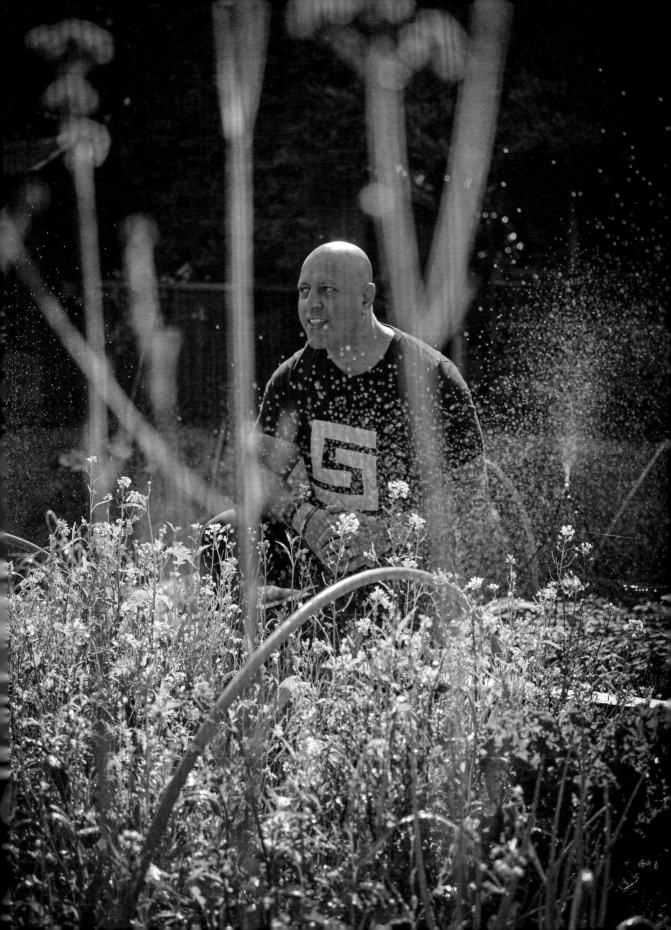

index

affogato with vanilla ice cream and olive oil 180–1

almonds
 cauliflower and almond soup 144–5
 my high-protein smoothie 160
 nut and seed crispy chicken escalope 118–19
 protein bar 184

amino acids 139, 156

anchovies 12
 baked courgettes, fennel seeds, olive oil and anchovies 70–1
 chicken meatballs with butter beans and lemon 124–5
 my spinach Caesar salad 46–7
 sirloin steak with my anchovy dressing 138–9

Angus's chimichurri 150–1

antioxidants 35, 42, 69, 79, 168, 183

apples
 crudités 40–1
 RSB overnight oats with seeds & nuts 174

Asian slaw 54–5

aubergines
 John's roast aubergine with harissa, chilli and pomegranate molasses 66–7
 Momma Bains' aubergine and potato sabji 68

bananas
 my high-protein smoothie 160
 porridge with nuts, seeds and fruit 172–3

barbecue potatoes with oregano, olive oil and goat's cheese 87

barley 19

basil
 pan-fried tuna marinated in soy, olive oil and basil 108
 triple-layered tomato, onion, fennel and basil salad 50–1

beans 19
 chicken meatballs with butter beans and lemon 124–5
 chunky venison chilli with bitter chocolate 134
 four-bean beef chilli 140–1
 my four-bean chilli 35
 my tuna Niçoise 56–7
 noodle and shaved vegetable salad 48–9

beef
 beef and lettuce burger 136–7
 my four-bean beef chilli 140–1
 sirloin steak with my anchovy dressing 138–9

beetroot, roasted beetroot with feta, mint and caraway seeds 86

beta-alanine 130

beta-carotene 17, 65

beta-glucan 19, 36, 173, 174

blueberries
 meringues with raspberries, blueberries and crème fraîche 178–9
 porridge with nuts, seeds and fruit 172–3

bone broth 157

broccoli, broccoli with spring onions, chilli, soy and sesame seeds 76, 95

Brussels sprouts
 Brussels sprout sabji 69
 stir-fried Brussels sprouts with cumin and cashews 78–9

burger, beef and lettuce 136–7

butternut squash, baked butternut squash, olive oil and Parmesan 88–9

cabbage
 kimchi 153
 my Asian slaw 54–5
 sauerkraut 154–5

capsaicin 147

carotenoids 166

carrots
 bone broth 157
 crudités 40–1
 my Asian slaw 54–5
 noodle and shaved vegetable salad 48–9
 oven-baked carrots with garam masala, mint, coriander, lime and yoghurt 64–5
 roasted root vegetables, rosemary, garlic and ras el hanout 72

cashew nuts
 oven-baked carrots with garam masala, mint, coriander, lime and yoghurt 64–5
 stir-fried Brussels sprouts with cumin and cashews 78–9

cauliflower
 cauliflower and almond soup 144–5
 Momma Bains' aloo gobi 82–3
 raw cauliflower salad 52–3, 127

cheese (cottage), flaked mackerel with scrambled egg and cottage cheese 96–7

cheese (feta)
 blended omelette with spinach and feta 30
 coddled eggs with caramelized onions and feta 26–7
 cubed potatoes with feta, olives and capers 84–5
 my Greek salad 42
 roasted beetroot with feta, mint and caraway seeds 86

cheese (goat's), barbecue potatoes with oregano, olive oil and goat's cheese 87

cheese (Parmesan) 12
  Angus's chimichurri 150-1
  baked butternut squash, olive oil
    and Parmesan 88-9
  baked salmon with wholemeal
    penne, lemon and rocket 92-3
  chicken meatballs with butter
    beans and lemon 124-5
  my spinach Caesar salad 46-7
chicken 14
  bone broth 157
  chicken meatballs with butter
    beans and lemon 124-5
  chicken with seven bulbs of garlic
    122-3
  minced chicken burger with ginger,
    garlic and baharat 120-1
  nut and seed crispy chicken
    escalope 118-19
  roast chicken salad, beluga lentils,
    pickled ginger and sriracha 58-9
  spatchcock chicken with roasted
    roots and herbs 116-17
chickpeas
  hummus 116, 162, 164-5
  Momma Bains' chickpea curry 62-3
chicory
  crudités 40-1
  my tuna Niçoise 56-7
chimichurri, Angus's 150-1
chocolate 14
  chocolate mousse with aged
    balsamic vinegar 182-3
  chocolate protein cookies 176
  chunky venison chilli with bitter
    chocolate 134, 169
  protein bar 184
cholesterol 17, 19, 20, 35, 169
  LDL 66, 70, 76
chorizo eggs with coriander 31
cod
  cod in baking parchment 94-5

cod with miso 54, 109
Sat's 'fishcakes' 110-11
coriander
  Angus's chimichurri 150-1
  chorizo eggs with coriander 31
  coriander salt 31
  mussels in white wine and
    coriander 98-9
  oven-baked carrots with garam
    masala, mint, coriander, lime
    and yoghurt 64-5
courgettes
  baked courgettes, fennel seeds,
    olive oil and anchovies 70-1
  noodle and shaved vegetable
    salad 48-9
crab 20
crudités 40-1, 165
cucumber
  chilled gazpacho with chilli 146-7
  crudités 40-1
  noodle and shaved vegetable
    salad 48-9

dashi 2, 14, 156

eggs 12, 22-37
  blended omelette with spinach
    and feta 30
  chocolate mousse with aged
    balsamic vinegar 182-3
  chorizo eggs with coriander 31
  coddled eggs with caramelized
    onions and feta 26-7
  flaked mackerel with scrambled
    egg and cottage cheese 96-7
  fried eggs in lots of olive oil and
    chilli (egg Banjo) 28-9
  leftover vegetable 'Spanish
    tortilla' 32-3
  my tuna Niçoise 56-7

pot-roast mushrooms with
    poached eggs and thyme 34-5
red pepper and onion frittata with
    tomato salsa 166-7
'Sat-Shuka' baked eggs with
    stewed leeks and chilli 24-5
shiitake mushrooms with beluga
    lentils and fried eggs 36-7
spinach and watercress soup
    148-9

fennel, triple-layered tomato, onion,
    fennel and basil salad 50-1
fermented foods 18, 153, 155
fibrous vegetables 18
fish 14, 90-113
  baked salmon with wholemeal
    penne, lemon and rocket 92-3
  cod in baking parchment 94-5
  cod with miso 54, 109
  flaked mackerel with scrambled
    egg and cottage cheese 96-7
  grilled salmon with pickled ginger
    and soy sauce 102-3
  mussels in white wine and
    coriander 98-9
  natural smoked haddock with
    preserved lemon and cumin
    100-1
  pan-fried tuna marinated in soy,
    olive oil and basil 108
  salmon XO 54, 104-5
  Sat's 'fishcakes' 110-11
  scallops cooked over open coals
    112-13
flatbreads
  potato flatbread 116, 127, 154, 162
  wholemeal flatbread 162
flavanols 183

garlic
 Angus's chimichurri 150-1
 chicken with seven bulbs of garlic
  122-3
 chilled gazpacho with chilli 146-7
 fried eggs in lots of olive oil and
  chilli (egg Banjo) 28-9
 kimchi 153
 minced chicken burger with ginger,
  garlic and baharat 120-1
ginger
 grilled salmon with pickled ginger
  and soy sauce 102-3
 kimchi 153
 roast chicken salad, beluga lentils,
  pickled ginger and sriracha 58-9
gingerol 95
glucosinolate 19
glutamate 12
glutathione 79
Greek salad 42
Greek yoghurt with strawberries,
 mint and olive oil 175
gut microbiome 19

hazelnuts, braised nuts 169
heart-healthy eating 16-21
herbs 20, 21
honey
 chocolate protein cookies 176
 Greek yoghurt with strawberries,
  mint and olive oil 175
 meringues with raspberries,
  blueberries and crème fraîche
  178-9
 my Asian slaw 54-5
 my high-protein smoothie 160
 olive oil shot 168
 RSB overnight oats with seeds &
  nuts 174
hummus 116, 162, 164-5

ice cream, affogato with vanilla ice
 cream and olive oil 180-1
iron 139

kaempferol 69
kimchi 153
 roast chicken salad, beluga lentils,
  pickled ginger and sriracha 58-9
koji 109
kombu seaweed 156

lamb
 dry-fried spiced lamb mince 126
 lamb chops with harissa 127
 my flattened lamb kofta/kebab
  53, 130-1, 162, 166
leeks
 bone broth 157
 'Sat-Shuka' baked eggs with
  stewed leeks and chilli 24-5
lemongrass, red lentil and
 lemongrass soup 152
lemons
 baked butternut squash, olive oil
  and Parmesan 88-9
 baked salmon with wholemeal
  penne, lemon and rocket 92-3
 chicken meatballs with butter
  beans and lemon 124-5
 lamb chops with harissa 127
 my spinach Caesar salad 46-7
 natural smoked haddock with
  preserved lemon and cumin
  100-1
 olive oil shot 168
lentils
 lentil dahl 72
 red lentil and lemongrass soup 152
 roast chicken salad, beluga lentils,
  pickled ginger and sriracha 58-9
 shiitake mushrooms with beluga
  lentils and fried eggs 36-7
lettuce
 beef and lettuce burger 136-7
 crudités 40-1
 dry-fried spiced lamb mince 126
limes
 Angus's chimichurri 150-1
 cod with miso 109

minced venison and oyster
 mushroom winter warmer 135
 my Asian slaw 54-5
 oven-baked carrots with garam
  masala, mint, coriander, lime
  and yoghurt 64-5
 raw cauliflower salad 52-3
lycopene 17, 65

mackerel, flaked mackerel with
 scrambled egg and cottage
 cheese 96-7
mangetout, noodle and shaved
 vegetable salad 48-9
meat 14, 20-1, 114-41
meringues with raspberries,
 blueberries and crème fraîche
 178-9
mint
 dry-fried spiced lamb mince 126
 Greek yoghurt with strawberries,
  mint and olive oil 175
 lamb chops with harissa 127
 my Punjabi salad 44-5
 oven-baked carrots with garam
  masala, mint, coriander, lime
  and yoghurt 64-5
 raw cauliflower salad 52-3
 roasted beetroot with feta, mint
  and caraway seeds 86
miso paste 109
Murphy, Mick 28
mushrooms
 minced venison and oyster
  mushroom winter warmer 135
 pot-roast mushrooms with
  poached eggs and thyme 34-5
 shiitake mushrooms with beluga
  lentils and fried eggs 36-7
mussels 20
 mussels in white wine and
  coriander 98-9

nasunin 66
nitrates 148

noodles, noodle and shaved vegetable salad 48-9
nuts 19
 braised nuts 169
 nut and seed crispy chicken escalope 118-19
 oven-baked carrots with garam masala, mint, coriander, lime and yoghurt 64-5
 porridge with nuts, seeds and fruit 172-3
 protein bar 184
 sirloin steak with my anchovy dressing 138-9
 stir-fried Brussels sprouts with cumin and cashews 78-9

oats 19
 protein bar 184
 RSB overnight oats with seeds & nuts 174
oily fish 14, 20
oligosaccharides 166
olive oil
 extra-virgin 19
 olive oil shot 168
olives
 cubed potatoes with feta, olives and capers 84-5
 my tuna Niçoise 56-7
omega-3 fatty acids 96, 99, 104, 108
onions (red)
 chilled gazpacho with chilli 146-7
 crudités 40-1
 my Greek salad 42
 my Punjabi salad 44-5
 my tuna Niçoise 56-7
 noodle and shaved vegetable salad 48-9
 red pepper and onion frittata with tomato salsa 166-7
 roasted root vegetables, rosemary, garlic and ras el hanout 72

triple-layered tomato, onion, fennel and basil salad 50-1
onions (white), coddled eggs with caramelized onions and feta 26-7

paneer, my Punjabi salad 44-5
parsnips, roasted root vegetables, rosemary, garlic and ras el hanout 72
pasta, baked salmon with wholemeal penne, lemon and rocket 92-3
peanut butter
 chocolate protein cookies 176
 my high-protein smoothie 160
 protein bar 184
pecan nuts, sirloin steak with my anchovy dressing 138-9
pectin 18, 87
peppers
 chilled gazpacho with chilli 146-7
 crudités 40-1
 my Asian slaw 54-5
 my four-bean beef chilli 140-1
 my tuna Niçoise 56-7
 red pepper and onion frittata with tomato salsa 166-7
phosphorus 95
pine nuts
 baked courgettes, fennel seeds, olive oil and anchovies 70-1
 baked salmon with wholemeal penne, lemon and rocket 92-3
 barbecue potatoes with oregano, olive oil and goat's cheese 87
 braised nuts 169
 hummus 116, 162, 164-5
 nut and seed crispy chicken escalope 118-19
pistachios
 braised nuts 169
 protein bar 184
polyphenols 151, 166, 183
pork, peppered pork chop with mustards 132-3

porridge with nuts, seeds and fruit 172-3
potatoes
 barbecue potatoes with oregano, olive oil and goat's cheese 87
 cubed potatoes with feta, olives and capers 84-5
 Momma Bains' aloo gobi 82-3
 Momma Bains' aubergine and potato sabji 68
 my tuna Niçoise 56-7
 potato flatbreads 116, 127, 154, 162
 roasted root vegetables, rosemary, garlic and ras el hanout 72
 Sat's 'fishcakes' 110-11
 spinach and watercress soup 148-9
prebiotics 18, 19, 183
probiotics 18, 109, 153
protein bar 184
pulses 19
Punjabi salad 44-5

raspberries
 meringues with raspberries, blueberries and crème fraîche 178-9
 porridge with nuts, seeds and fruit 172-3
rocket, baked salmon with wholemeal penne, lemon and rocket 92-3
RSB overnight oats with seeds & nuts 174

salads 13, 38-59
 crudités 40-1
 my Asian slaw 54-5
 my Greek salad 42
 my Punjabi salad 44-5
 my spinach Caesar salad 46-7
 my tuna Niçoise 56-7
 my warm spinach salad 43

raw cauliflower salad 52-3
roast chicken salad, beluga lentils,
    pickled ginger and sriracha 58-9
triple-layered tomato, onion,
    fennel and basil salad 50-1
salmon
    baked salmon with wholemeal
        penne, lemon and rocket 92-3
    grilled salmon with pickled ginger
        and soy sauce 102-3
    salmon XO 54, 104-5
'Sat-Shuka' baked eggs with stewed
    leeks and chilli 24-5
sauerkraut 154-5
seeds 19
    my Asian slaw 54-5
    noodle and shaved vegetable
        salad 48-9
    nut and seed crispy chicken
        escalope 118-19
    porridge with nuts, seeds and fruit
        172-3
    RSB overnight oats with seeds &
        nuts 174
selenium 95, 96, 112
shellfish 20
shiitake mushrooms with beluga
    lentils and fried eggs 36-7
smoked fish
    natural smoked haddock with
        preserved lemon and cumin
        100-1
    Sat's 'fishcakes' 110-11
smoothies 160, 161
soluble fibre 18, 19, 87
soups 14
    bone broth 157
    cauliflower and almond soup
        144-5
    chilled gazpacho with chilli 146-7
    red lentil and lemongrass soup
        152
    spinach and watercress soup
        148-9
spices 20, 21

spinach
    blended omelette with spinach
        and feta 30
    my spinach Caesar salad 46-7
    my warm spinach salad 43
    'Sat-Shuka' baked eggs with
        stewed leeks and chilli 24-5
    spinach and almond smoothie 161
    spinach and watercress soup
        148-9
strawberries
    Greek yoghurt with strawberries,
        mint and olive oil 175
    porridge with nuts, seeds and fruit
        172-3
sulforaphane 53, 76
sweet potatoes, spiced sweet
    potato fries 80-1

thiamine 133
tomatoes
    chilled gazpacho with chilli 146-7
    Momma Bains' aloo gobi 82-3
    my Greek salad 42
    my Punjabi salad 44-5
    my tuna Niçoise 56-7
    red pepper and onion frittata with
        tomato salsa 166-7
    triple-layered tomato, onion,
        fennel and basil salad 50-1
tomatoes (tinned)
    Brussels sprout sabji 69
    chicken meatballs with butter
        beans and lemon 124-5
    Momma Bains' aubergine and
        potato sabji 68
    Momma Bains' chickpea curry 62-3
triglycerides 108
tuna
    my tuna Niçoise 56-7
    pan-fried tuna marinated in soy,
        olive oil and basil 108

umami 12, 156

vegetables 18, 60-89
    crudités 40-1
    leftover vegetable 'Spanish
        tortilla' 32-3
    noodle and shaved vegetable
        salad 48-9
    roasted root vegetables,
        rosemary, garlic and ras el
        hanout 72
    spatchcock chicken with roasted
        roots and herbs 116-17
venison
    chunky venison chilli with bitter
        chocolate 134, 169
    minced venison and oyster
        mushroom winter warmer 135
vitamin B12 100, 133
vitamin K 148

watercress, spinach and watercress
    soup 148-9

XO sauce 104-5

yoghurt
    dry-fried spiced lamb mince 126
    Greek yoghurt with strawberries,
        mint and olive oil 175
    oven-baked carrots with garam
        masala, mint, coriander, lime
        and yoghurt 64-5
    RSB overnight oats with seeds &
        nuts 174

zinc 112, 133

acknowledgements

Writing a book like this relies on a tremendous amount of help and support from behind the scenes. I would like to thank the people that have helped me during this chapter of my life, including:

My whole team at RSB for allowing me to use them as guinea pigs for recipe testing, especially the front of house team, as they aren't professionally trained chefs. It was the perfect opportunity to replicate the way someone at home would cook and has, I believe, made the recipes even more attainable for you, ironing out any cooking, weights and practical issues.

My family and friends that helped me in my recovery, I will always be indebted to you.

My agent, Borra and her team at DML Talent for their insight and support on working on a project like this and for being at the end of the phone for all my queries.
Judith Hannam and her whole team at Kyle Books who believed there was good reason for a book like this to exist and allowed me to learn a whole new side to cooking at home and menu writing.

The food stylist, Katie Marshall. Wow, I have a new appreciation for the work that goes on behind the scenes of creating beautiful images!

Jodi Hinds, the best photographer I have worked with, for making the food look so incredible and delicious.

The doctors, nurses and rehab team that looked after me at Nottingham City Hospital

My surgeon, Mr Naik, for giving me the best possible chance for a healthy, 'normal' life with his life-saving surgical skills.

Dr Richard Varcoe, Consultant Interventional Cardiologist at Nottingham University Hospital NHS Trust, for his support, advice, incredible after care and regular checkups making sure I am on track.

Dr Neil Williams, Senior Lecturer in Exercise Physiology and Nutrition at Nottingham Trent University, whose eye for detail, knowledge and support on this project were such a positive that I knew he was the man for the job. Neil was one of the first people I reached out to whilst in hospital, as I knew the key to my recovery lay in food and nutrition. My insight into the benefit of ingredients since writing this book has increased beyond recognition and that is thanks to Neil. The information he has shared is insightful and easy to understand, and I know will help you when creating the recipes.

John Freeman, my Head Chef for over 20 years, for his support, professionalism, incredible eye for detail, and for making sure each recipe was water tight, tried and tested. His running of the kitchen whilst I was writing and shooting allowed me to give my full concentration to this book.
Thank you, John. x

Amanda Bains, my incredible wife, for her uncompromising, unconditional love, for her patience, strength and resolve. These are only a few of the adjectives I could use. Without her I would not be as strong as I am today. She makes me want to share as many new experiences and memories with her and has created a new perspective on life. We hear all the time that 'life is short, make the most of it'. I believe that more than ever now and want to thank Amanda from the bottom of my mended heart. 🖤 🩹
I love You xxxxxxx = 7

Lastly, to the two cutest loving rabbits I have:
Winter and Minty. They make every day that bit better.
🐾 🐾 🖤

An Hachette UK Company
www.hachette.co.uk

First published in Great Britain in 2024 by
Kyle Books, an imprint of Octopus Publishing Group Limited
Carmelite House
50 Victoria Embankment
London EC4Y 0DZ
www.octopusbooks.co.uk

ISBN: 9781804190722

Distributed in the US by Hachette Book Group, 1290 Avenue
of the Americas, 4th and 5th Floors, New York, NY 10104

Distributed in Canada by Canadian Manda Group,
664 Annette St., Toronto, Ontario, Canada M6S 2C8

Publishing Director: Judith Hannam
Publisher: Joanna Copestick
Project Editor: Samhita Foria
Design: Paul Palmer-Edwards
Cover Design: Yasia Williams
Food styling: Katie Marshall
Props styling: Lydia McPherson
Production: Lisa Pinnell

Printed and bound in China

10 9 8 7 6 5 4 3 2 1

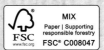

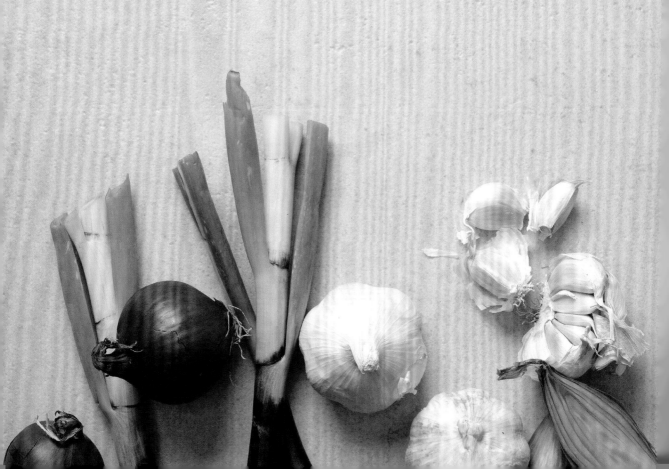